THE DATTOLI BLUE RIBBON PROSTATE CANCER SOLUTION

HOW TO SURVIVE AND THRIVE WITHOUT SURGERY

THE DATTOLI BLUE RIBBON PROSTATE CANCER SOLUTION

HOW TO SURVIVE AND THRIVE WITHOUT SURGERY

MICHAEL J. DATTOLI, MD

JENNIFER CASH, ARNP, MS, OCN

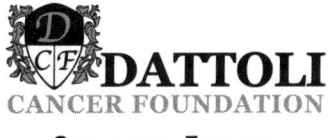

DATTOLI
CANCER FOUNDATION

SARASOTA, FLORIDA

Published by the Dattoli Cancer Foundation

ISBN-10: 0979468094
ISBN-13: 9780979468094

Library of Congress Control Number: Pending

For information on distributor to the trade in the United States, contact:
Dattoli Cancer Foundation, 2803 Fruitville Road, Sarasota, FL 34237 (800-915-1001)

Book design and composition by Design Corps, Batavia, IL

Printed by Marrakesh Express, Tarpon Springs, Florida

DEDICATION

This book is dedicated to all those whose lives have been touched by prostate cancer, and to the patients and their families whom we are privileged to serve and educate as cancer care providers.

MEDICAL DISCLAIMER

ACKNOWLEDGMENTS

We are indebted to a number of members of the Dattoli Team who have contributed to this book: Greg Lawrence for his editorial efforts, Dawn Horowitz-Toscano, Ginya Carnahan, Meg Brockett, Chris Wells, Jone Fay, RT, CMD, Jennifer Hogan, MLT, ASCP, and Jack Crowley of the Dattoli Cancer Center & Brachytherapy Research Institute for their contributions and ongoing support.

We are deeply grateful to all the wonderful patients and family members who have turned to the Dattoli Cancer Foundation for counseling and guidance and in turn have given us their encouragement and support. It is your spirit and commitment in confronting this disease that inspires us all, and enables us to fulfill our mission.

CONTENTS

Part One—The Non-Surgical Approach to Diagnosis and Treatment

by Michael Dattoli, M.D.

Part Two—Post-treatment Care and Lifestyle Changes

by Jennifer Cash, ARNP, MS, OCN®

Appendices

THE ESSENTIAL TOOLS FOR FIGHTING PROSTATE CANCER

BY MICHAEL J. DATTOLI, M.D.

Having spent more than twenty five years studying prostate cancer and treating more than ten thousand men, I am well aware of the controversies in this field of medicine, including when to treat and when not to treat this disease. Many Americans don't know that with the exception of skin cancers, prostate cancer is today's most commonly diagnosed cancer, even surpassing breast cancer. The good news is that unlike other cancers, such as lung cancer or colon cancer, prostate cancer is typically more curable.

While we are learning more each day, there are still unsolved mysteries and many conflicting viewpoints about this disease. Some prostate cancers are rather indolent and slow-growing and may not require treatment, while others are rapidly spreading and potentially lethal, usually calling for some form of treatment. Some prostate cancer tumors make themselves known by driving up prostatic specific antigen (PSA) levels in the blood, while others lurk in the gland without raising the PSA red flag and can only be identified through skilled digital examination and highly sophisticated technologies such as color-flow Doppler ultrasound. Determining which prostate cancers are aggressive and life-threatening is crucial in deciding which patients should be treated.

What is a man to do in the face of the ongoing debates as to the value of PSA screening? My advice is to heed the recommendations of the American Cancer Society, the National Cancer Institute, and other mainstream organizations addressing prostate cancer issues: Consult your personal physician and consider having an annual prostate exam by a board-certified internist or urologist, beginning at age 50 (age 45 or earlier if there is a family history of prostate cancer or if the man is African-American). The exam should include both the PSA blood test and a digital rectal exam.

If your doctor suspects you may have prostate cancer, the only way to be sure is by undergoing a prostate biopsy and having a pathologist examine tissue samples. Make sure your doctor takes at least 12 core samples in the biopsy–the more samples, the better your chance will be of obtaining an accurate result. With regard to diagnosis and treatment, it is often wise to obtain second opinions from one or more specialists within the field, keeping in mind that each specialist is likely to be biased to some degree toward his or her own particular treatment specialty.

If you are diagnosed with prostate cancer, give yourself time to evaluate ALL your treatment options. Don't make a panicked, knee-jerk decision while still in the shock of hearing your diagnosis. We are fortunate to live at a time when there are a number of effective treatment options for this disease. Some of these, such as brachytherapy (pronounced brăk-ē-therapy) and 4-Dimensional Image-Guided Intensity Modulated Radiation Therapy (4D IG-IMRT)–are relatively noninvasive and have profoundly improved our ability to maintain quality of life for patients. In addition, thanks to these therapeutic innovations, we are now able to successfully treat even high risk patients (those with high PSA values, high Gleason scores, and locally advanced cancer).

As you investigate your treatment options, depending on the specifics of your case, weigh the pros and cons of each type of therapy for which you are a candidate. And ask your doctor the hard questions about any treatment you may consider: How many men have you treated with this therapy? How many have a profile similar to mine? What are the published success rates of this therapy? What are your success rates? It is also wise to seek out other men who have been treated for prostate cancer. You may benefit by attending one of the Man-to-Man support group meetings sponsored by the American Cancer Society, or Us TOO International meetings. By gathering all of the relevant facts that you can, you will be able to make a more fully informed treatment decision.

I strongly encourage you to work with your doctor and become an integral part of that decision-making process. As you conduct your research, be cautious about what you read in the news media, and consider the sources. There are many misconceptions about prostate cancer that find their way into the media, including many of the popular medical websites and blogs on the Internet. Remember that just because something is "new" doesn't mean it is better or has been proven to be effective. You will want to place your confidence—and your life and quality of life after treatment—in the hands of an experienced physician who can show you his or her long-term track record.

In my practice, which is entirely devoted to prostate cancer, I want my patients to be very comfortable with their treatment. The patient who has become informed and knows what to anticipate will come through his treatment with more practical knowledge and greater peace of mind.

Sometimes I can tell that a man is not going to be comfortable with any treatment other than one of the surgical options. Some men have that mindset. When I sense that is the case, I may tell him that if his test results predict that his cancer is still confined to the prostate gland, perhaps he can indeed undergo surgery if he is so inclined. In discussing treatment options with patients, I try to be as even-keeled as possible, knowing that the choice is ultimately theirs to make. At the same time, I want each patient to be aware as much as possible of the peer-reviewed results published in the field by the leading practitioners of each type of treatment.

I find that the data often speaks for itself. While it may sound very logical to say, "You have a cancer, and we should cut it out," this option may not be so attractive if the patient is also told that even in the best surgical hands, there is a high probability that some cancer will be left behind after surgery, that there is a risk he may have to wear diapers for the rest of his life, and there is a strong likelihood that he will suffer from erectile dysfunction. Armed with this additional information based on the most recent surgical data, the patient may want to think very hard about his choice and at least consider other options. In the end, whatever he decides, each man should feel confident that he has made the right choice for himself based on his own particular needs and individual case.

The purpose of this book is to provide you with the most up to date and accurate information to help guide you from diagnosis to recovery. Before making any decisions about treatment, you should carefully evaluate the likelihood of cure for each treatment option and the risk of side effects that may alter your quality of life. Taking into account your age, overall health, and the extent and aggressiveness of the cancer, you will want to find a balance between treatment effectiveness and potential side effects—a balance with which you are comfortable and can live with before, during and after treatment. Regardless of the type of therapy you decide is right for you, having a positive mental outlook and knowing what to expect each step of the way are keys to winning the fight against this disease.

PART ONE

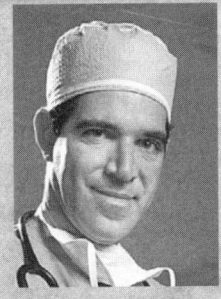

BY MICHAEL DATTOLI, M.D

The entire field of prostate cancer diagnosis and treatment has undergone a revolution during the past few decades, in part brought about by widespread screening with the PSA blood test, which has allowed for earlier diagnosis of the disease. We have also seen dramatic technological progress in each of the medical specialties that are involved in the field. All of these changes have improved the prognosis for most patients regardless of their age and the stage of their cancers.

THE NON-SURGICAL APPROACH TO DIAGNOSIS AND TREATMENT

Recent advances in the delivery of high energy photons, ultrasound imaging, and computerized treatment planning have essentially turned the tide against what was previously thought to be a disease most effectively treated by means of radical surgery. At this time, an overview of prostate cancer care and treatment from a non-surgical perspective, as presented in this book, is crucial for every patient wishing to receive the highest standard of care. The discussion that follows is intended to provide the latest data and essential knowledge to prepare patients to make fully informed decisions about their treatment options with their doctors.

CHAPTER ONE

THE BASICS OF PROSTATE CANCER

What is prostate cancer?

Prostate cancer (PCa) is the most commonly diagnosed cancer in men. Since the advent of screening with the PSA blood test in the late 1980s, prostate cancer has been diagnosed more frequently, reaching epidemic proportions during the last decade. It is second only to lung cancer as a leading cause of cancer death in the male population. That grim statistic, however, is likely to change as the disease is increasingly diagnosed earlier when it is more treatable.

Where is the Prostate Gland Located and what is its Function?

The prostate is a walnut-size gland located at the bottom of the pelvis, just beneath the bladder and in front of the rectum (see Figure 1). Found only in men, the prostate gland surrounds an approximate inch-long segment of the urethra, the channel through which urine exits the bladder and passes out of the body. The primary function of the prostate is to produce some of the seminal fluid, which flows into the urethra at the time of orgasm. The fluid allows for nourishment and transport of the sperm at ejaculation. The seminal vesicles are two sac-like structures that are attached to the back of the prostate and produce additional seminal fluid that passes through the gland. At the time of orgasm, the prostate mechanically contracts to propel the ejaculate towards the penis.

The prostate gland contains many hundreds of tiny passageways lined with cells that produce seminal fluid. Normally, these lining cells reproduce

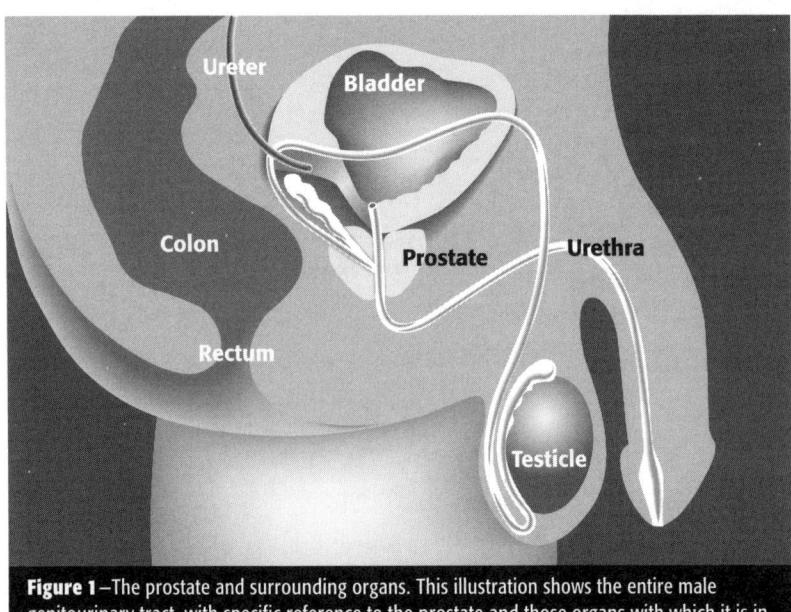

Figure 1—The prostate and surrounding organs. This illustration shows the entire male genitourinary tract, with specific reference to the prostate and those organs with which it is in close relationship.

slowly, at about the same rate that cells die. But with cancer, some of these cells become abnormal and reproduce at an uncontrollable rate. Although several other cell types are found in the prostate, more than 99% of prostate cancers develop from the glandular cells. The medical term for cancer that starts in glandular cells like these is *adenocarcinoma.* Over time, the build-up of cancerous cells in the gland produces a lump or "tumor." By the time a tumor is palpable, at least a billion cells are present.

The location of the prostate makes the whole issue of diagnosing and treating prostate cancer very challenging. The prostate is down in the well of the pelvis, with a lot of nerves and arteries going to the gland. It's one of the most difficult locations in the body to get at because it's entangled by a web of vessels and nerves. and surrounded by critical organs, including but not limited to the bladder, rectum, internal and external sphincters, and the large neurovascular bundles on the right and left side of the gland. This makes all therapies challenging, and that's why many patients will have a prolonged procedure with surgery, and even with newer modalities such as laparoscopic and robotic surgery. It can become a far more complicated procedure if one of these vessels is nicked.

The problem with prostate cancer tends to be the location where most cancers begin, which is the periphery of the gland. This is the peripheral zone. The vast majority of cancers begin there—depending on the study you read, 70% to 95%. That's not to say that they can't occur elsewhere, but if they do occur in the central zone for example, it's not such an issue. Those tend to be clinically insignificant. It's the cancers that occur at the posterior boundary that present most of the problems.

It should be noted that prostate cancer is not contagious. Nor can it be sexually transmitted. Because prostate cancer grows so slowly, it often causes no symptoms in the early stages. When symptoms do occur, they usually take the form of difficult or frequent urination, a slow or weak urine stream and/or urination during the night (nocturia). These same symptoms, however, are more often caused by an overgrowth of normal prostate tissue that commonly occurs with aging. This non-cancerous condition is known as benign prostatic hypertrophy, or BPH (See Figure 2).

Although many men with BPH never experience serious problems due to the condition, with sufficient time, symptoms will begin to manifest. As the prostate gland enlarges, BPH tissue may constrict the urethra. There are a variety of medications that can be prescribed to treat the symptoms of BPH, including alpha-blockers such as Hytrin®, Cardura®, Flomax® and

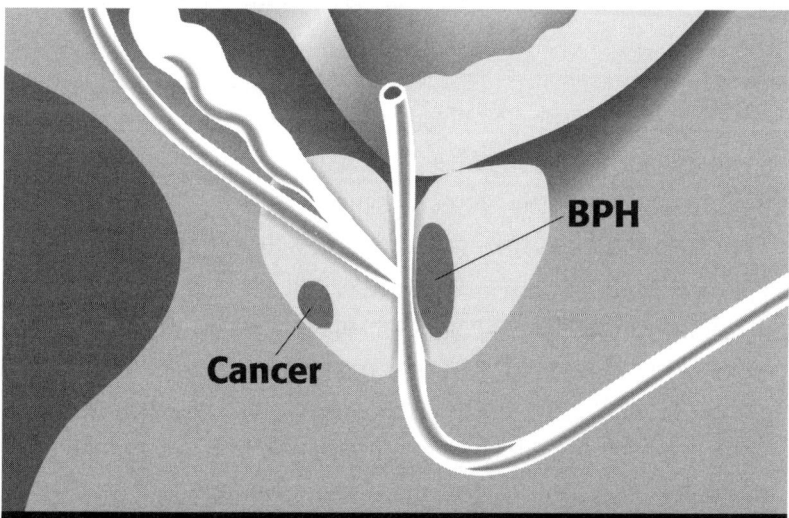

Figure 2–A prostate gland showing both BPH and cancer. BPH usually begins near the core, while prostate cancer more often arises near the boundary of the gland.

Uroxatral®, and agents that interfere with the production of dihydrotestosterone, such as Proscar® (finasteride) and Avodart®. None of these medications are to be considered treatments for prostate cancer, but only to ameliorate symptoms caused by BPH or prostate cancer.

The most common surgical approach to BPH is called a transurethral resection of the prostate (TURP), a procedure which involves the use of a surgical instrument to trim BPH tissue from the tip of the prostate gland where it meets the bladder from within the prostatic urethra. This has been traditionally a resectoscope, although laser procedures are gaining increasing popularity (e.g. Holmium, SLV and Green Light lasers). Other treatment methods take advantage of the fact that heat (thermopathy) eradicates benign cells (e.g. the indigo laser or the Targis™ microwave system). If the prostate is extremely enlarged, an open surgical procedure known as a simple prostatectomy may be indicated. The latter procedure was the most common performed before 1970 and is rarely performed today.

How Common is Prostate Cancer?

The American Cancer Society (ACS) estimates that in 2008 approximately 186,320 men will be diagnosed with prostate cancer in the U.S. and about 28,660 men will die from the disease, making it the second leading cause of cancer death in men after lung cancer. As noted, since the late 1980s, prostate cancer incidence rates have increased significantly because the prostate-specific antigen (PSA) blood test has allowed for earlier diagnosis in men without symptoms. While the disease is being diagnosed earlier, the death rate for prostate cancer is going down.

Prostate cancer becomes more prevalent with age. More than 70% of all prostate cancer cases are diagnosed in patients over age 65. Because the U.S. has a rapidly aging population, the problem is on the rise. Many physicians are also seeing a growing number of younger patients, from 30 to 65. Whether this is due to earlier screening and detection or disease migration to younger individuals is currently unknown. In view of the fact that most younger patients have more aggressive cancers, it is unlikely a function of earlier screening (most present with symptoms or abnormal digital rectal exams).

Prostate cancer may exist in combination with benign conditions, such as BPH. Since the symptoms of prostate cancer (see below) resemble or are in some cases identical with symptoms for benign conditions, appropriate diagnostic tests must be performed to make an accurate diagnosis.

What Causes Prostate Cancer?

The exact causes of prostate cancer are unknown, but a combination of genetic and environmental factors, including certain aspects of the lifestyle in western countries, probably contributes to the progression of the disease. Researchers have identified several inherited genes that appear to increase the risk of prostate cancer. We know that at least 10% of prostate cancers are inherited directly from parents, while most prostate cancers appear to be acquired because of the way we live and what we are exposed to in the environment. These non-genetic factors may include diet, smoking, industrial pollution, excessive alcohol consumption, association with certain viruses (e.g. human papilloma virus), stress, and so forth.

Symptoms of Prostate Cancer*

✔ Blood in urine (hematuria).
✔ Pain or difficulty urinating.
✔ Increased frequency of urination, often at night (nocturia).
✔ Increased voiding urgency.
✔ Hesitant or intermittent urinary flow.
✔ Inability to urinate.
✔ Pain or discomfort in area of prostate.
✔ Trouble having or keeping an erection (erectile dysfunction).
✔ Weakness or numbness in the legs or feet.
✔ Unusual and unexplained weight loss.
✔ Continual pain in bones of lower back, hips or pelvis.

* All symtoms listed may be due to benign conditions of the prostate, or other conditions entirely unrelated to prostate cancer. Weakness or numbness in the lower extremities, for example, would not only be a symptom of far advanced prostate cancer with spread to the spine but a symptom of virtually any advanced malignancy, as well as other conditions.

Autopsy studies have shown that even in men over the age of 30, about a third will have microscopic prostate cancer regardless of their geographical location. Most, however, are low grade tumors. There is a gross discrepancy between the high rate of clinical prostate cancer in the U.S. and Western Europe compared to that in Asian countries like Japan. So it would seem there is something that keeps the microscopic cancer localized in Asian men, while the cancer is not contained in Western men. This finding is strengthened by studies showing that for Asian men who migrate to the U.S., the incidence of clinical prostate cancer increases up to seven times in one generation. One factor that researchers believe may account for the geographical discrepancy with prostate cancer is diet, especially, the higher intake of saturated fat and red meat in the U.S. and Western Europe compared to Asia.

While much about the manner in which cancer begins and proliferates remains mysterious, one thing is clear: damage to a critical portion of the cell's genetic code must occur for the cell to become cancerous. The cancer cell then replicates itself by division, and produces new generations of altered cells, bearing the genetic errors that produce cancer.

The genetic code for human beings is about three billion "letters" long, and is reproduced in every cell in the body. This code is broken up among hundreds of thousands of genes. Damaged cancer-causing genes have been given the name oncogenes, a combination of the Greek root onco, meaning "tumor," and gene. The discovery of oncogenes in the 1970s opened up new vistas of scientific exploration into cancer and its causes.

Not every gene has the potential to become an oncogene. Those genes that can by random error be transformed into cancer-causing genes are called proto-oncogenes. They are typically involved in the signaling mechanisms that control cellular growth and differentiation. Researchers have isolated dozens of these proto-oncogenes. It has been found that some oncogenes, such as an oncogene in bladder cancer, differ from the normal, functioning genes by only a single "letter" in the genetic code. There are several different means under investigation by which proto-oncogenes may become cancer genes. These include:

➤ Mutations caused by some outside agent, such as contact with a carcinogen, such as cigarette smoke or dietary carcinogens.

➤ Gene amplification, which is the production of too many copies of the same gene.

➤ Chromosomal translocation, or the rearrangement of genes.

Several oncogenes may be involved in the development of a particular kind of cancer. It has been estimated that ten to fifteen genetic changes may be required to develop lung cancer. Research is underway to identify those oncogenes involved in the development of prostate cancer as well. Researchers hope that once the mechanisms that produce prostate cancer are known, they can be counteracted on a molecular level.

The emergence of a cancer cell somewhere in the body does not mean that cancer will persist and proliferate. Many cancers are destroyed by the immune system before a serious malignancy can develop. This has been identified when patients undergo initial biopsies (e.g. breast and prostate) at which time special assays known as RT-PCR (reverse transcription polymerase chain reaction) have documented the presence of cancer cells in the blood at 80%. Many of these patients clearly do not go on to develop the disease. Why the immune system successfully counteracts the development of these abnormal cells in some instances and fails in others is a matter of speculation.

Some researchers suggest the immune system must be weakened or altered before an early cancer can advance. This has led to a new avenue of cancer research which seeks to fortify the immune system, called immunotherapy.

The discovery of the tumor-suppressor gene has also become the focus of much attention. When functioning properly, the tumor-suppressor gene will sense abnormal cell growth, and activate, causing the offending cells to die. Failure of this gene may also be involved in the inability of the body to control malignant growth.

Who is Most at Risk for Prostate Cancer?

Age, race and family history are the most important risk factors for prostate cancer. Those men who are most at risk are those with a positive family history, Caucasians 50 years of age or older, and African American males over 40 years of age. Prostate cancer occurs almost 70% more often in African-

American men than it does in white American men, and African Americans have the highest prostate cancer mortality rates of any ethnic group.

Studies also indicate that men with a family history of the disease are two or three times more likely to get prostate cancer. The likelihood that a man will inherit the disease increases if 1) two generations of his family have had prostate cancer, 2) two or more immediate relatives have had prostate cancer (brothers and/or father), and 3) one or more relatives are diagnosed before the age of 55.

What Types of Doctors Treat Prostate Cancer?

The treatment of prostate cancer is divided between several medical specialties: urologists (surgeons), radiation oncologists, and more recently, medical oncologists (chemotherapists). Urologists are doctors who spend one year after medical school studying general surgery, and three additional years studying surgical treatment of the sexual organs and urinary tract. Radiation oncologists are doctors who spend one to three years after medical school studying general medicine and four additional years studying the use of radiation for treating all types of cancer. Medical oncologists spend three years after medical school studying internal medicine and two additional years studying the use of chemotherapy, and to a lesser degree studying hormonal therapies. All of the disciplines may pursue further training called a "fellowship" in a chosen specialty.

In many cases, the specialties overlap. Urologists sometimes perform radioactive seed implants, although it is mandatory that they utilize a qualified radiation oncologist in order to treat with radiation. Some radiation oncologists perform the procedure without the aid of a urologist. Both urologists and radiation oncologists often prescribe hormonal therapy, as do medical oncologists. Most newly diagnosed patients are first referred by their personal physician to a urologist, and are often encouraged to have surgical treatment before they have had the opportunity to fully assess their other options. For this reason, patients are well advised not to rush into any form of treatment, to do their own research and obtain second opinions from the other specialties. It should be noted that in most states women having breast cancer are mandated to see both a surgeon and an oncologist. This is not yet the case with prostate cancer, though patients diagnosed with prostate cancer are well advised to consult both the surgical and radiation oncology specialists to understand their full range of treatment options.

Why is the Treatment of Prostate Cancer so Controversial?

Part of the reason this field is controversial is due to the fact that regardless of which treatment is used, patients have a reasonable, short-term, disease-free prognosis, which is unlike most other cancers. This is true even for prostate cancer patients who undergo the more esoteric or investigational therapies (e.g. cyberknife and HIFU, as discussed in later chapters). Even patients who choose not to be treated are most likely not going to die in the short term. In addition, when a primary therapy like radiation or surgery fails, there are other treatments like hormonal therapy or other systemic medications to fall back on. This is a different kind of situation than you find with most other diseases.

With other cancers, you're really put in a position where your back is against the wall and you're fighting for your life. As a doctor, you're in the fifteenth round, and you have to knock this cancer out, or that's it for your patient. This may also be the case with some aggressive prostate cancers. With this disease, we have a variety of specialties, all of which offer treatments that can potentially knock the cancer out at least for a while. In this situation, each type of specialist can argue that the specialty he has been trained in and practices offers the best therapy. Despite the fact that prostate cancer can be controlled in the short run, it is actually a very difficult cancer to "cure."

In order for you as a patient to find your way through these conflicting viewpoints, a careful evaluation of the latest data on cure rates and quality of life is essential to consider along with the specifics of your case and your individual needs. This is especially important since despite the relatively slow growth of most prostate cancers, relapse may follow a slow, painful course. Many doctors believe that progressive prostate cancer is the worst type of cancer because it kills you slowly!

The argument over which type of treatment is best continues because there are no definitive randomized trials that would definitively compare the various specialties and the different treatments they offer. However, what we can do is rigorously compare the results obtained by the premier treatment centers for each specialty and each type of treatment. That type of comparison is available to both doctors and patients and probably explains why the trend is moving away from surgery, with an increasing number of patients choosing one or more forms radiation therapy.

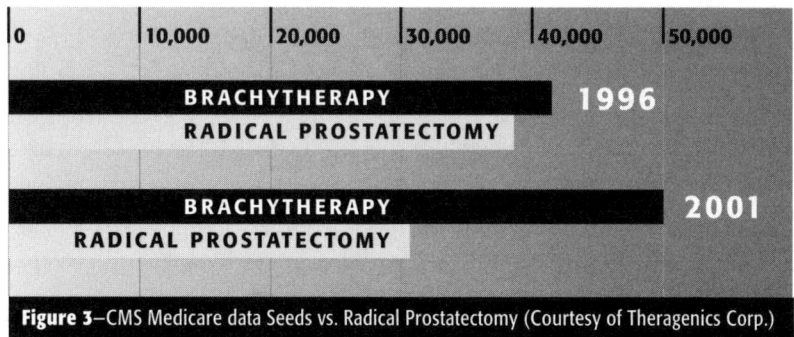

Figure 3–CMS Medicare data Seeds vs. Radical Prostatectomy (Courtesy of Theragenics Corp.)

How Do You Find the Doctor Who is Right For You?

A number of criteria can be used to help you evaluate a doctor's merit. A doctor with staff privileges at one or more hospitals will have usually demonstrated the necessary proficiency in his field to earn the respect of his or her colleagues. Review-committee membership at a respected medical institution also indicates a doctor's reputation among peers. A doctor whose practice is hospital-based or part of a group practice may be preferred, since any reputable hospital or group practice will require their physicians to undergo peer review sufficient to ensure quality care.

It is advisable to find a doctor who treats a large number of prostate cancer patients, and is therefore more familiar with the kind of care they require. Board certification will indicate that a doctor has been thoroughly examined although it cannot guarantee his competence. Certification in a specialty, especially oncology, or possession of a board fellowship are further indications of distinction. It is possible to check the credentials of a doctor with the Directory of Medical Specialists or the American Medical Directory, a copy of which can usually be found in the reference room of your local library. You might also ask a doctor for his or her curriculum vitae.

Any of these criteria will improve your chances of finding a capable physician. You might start as many patients do with a referral from a local, trusted doctor who is familiar with the reputable and respected physicians in your area. Keep in mind, however, that most general practitioners typically know very little about prostate cancer, and have historically referred prostate cancer patients to a urologist, who is likely to recommend surgical treatment rather than one of the non-surgical options.

A good physician will explain your condition in detail, taking the time to answer all of your questions and correcting any misconceptions you may have. It is your right to receive a complete description of all your options, and their advantages and disadvantages. This is vital information if you are to have a sense of control over what is happening to you. If the doctor fails to disclose this information, or does not encourage you to choose for yourself which treatment you wish to receive, find another doctor.

Throughout the period of your treatment, the physician should continue to keep you fully informed of the nature and rationale behind any tests or procedures recommended to you. Clear and concise written materials that explain the basic facts of prostate cancer, its symptoms and all of your treatment options, should also be made available to you.

A doctor who communicates concern for the patient as an individual can ease the treatment process. A physician who cares is more likely to inspire trust in his patients and help to allay their fears. But a doctor who sees each patient only as another medical condition to treat will most likely leave his patients feeling alienated, confused and anxious. Ultimately, such a doctor will impede the progress of those under his care.

In the final analysis, you need to have a comfort level with your doctor that enables to you answer the following questions affirmatively. Do you trust and have confidence in your doctor? Does he put you at ease? Are you able to talk with your doctor in a relaxed manner? Does he publish his results in reputable medical journals, or does he simply tell you that his patients "do fine" with his treatment? Is he forthcoming with you about his data?

A physician may be completely suited for treating some patients and unsuited for treating others. It may be nothing more than a matter of incompatible personalities. But you will be making critical decisions with this doctor, and undergoing a treatment process that can be difficult and extend for months or even years. Is the physician only interested in treating you, or will he follow you after treatment annually or biannually? You will need a doctor you can depend on when the going gets tough. If for any reason you do not feel comfortable with your physician, you should carefully consider whether it is in your interests to find care elsewhere.

When Should Prostate Cancer not be Treated?

Studies have shown that with early stage prostate cancer patients who are not treated, the risk of dying from the disease is very low for the first 10 years after diagnosis. Therefore, in the past, it was argued that prostate cancer patients with a life expectancy of less than 10 years should not be treated, because they were more likely to die from some other cause. With life expectancy increasing for the population as a whole, there are actually fewer and fewer cases of prostate cancer these days that do not call for some form of treatment, and the relatively non-invasive therapies such as brachytherapy and/or IMRT are often appropriate for older men who are otherwise in good health.

According to the most recent actuarial data, a 60-year-old man has a life expectancy of 21.1 years. He should therefore pursue some form of treatment because he will probably live long enough to die from his prostate cancer if it isn't treated. Even an 80-year-old man now has a life expectancy of 8.3 years. In the case of an 80-year-old whose general health is good and who has no other serious health conditions, he too stands a good chance of living beyond 10 years and would also be wise to consider treatment (see additional discussion below regarding screening, treatment and life expectancy).

What is "Watchful Waiting" and when is it Recommended?

Watchful waiting, or expectant surveillance, is an option for some early stage prostate cancer patients who want to try to preserve their quality of life by avoiding aggressive treatment for their cancer at least temporarily. These men may be advised to wait and monitor the progression of their cancer with periodic laboratory tests and physical examinations. Although I inform my patients of this option, I'm generally opposed to it for most men, because I don't see much merit to the idea of waiting as cancer progresses and becomes less treatable. Nor do I see much data to support this approach. The exceptions are those patients regardless of age who have a life expectancy less than ten years because of some other significant medical condition, such as heart disease or another form of cancer that is likely to be a cause of death before prostate cancer. For these men, watchful waiting may be a more realistic option.

Advocates of watchful waiting often correctly point out that the term is misleading and should not imply passive waiting or doing nothing. A more active program of surveillance is intended and may include a diet and fitness regimen undertaken in consultation with a doctor and tailored to the patient's condition. The process of waiting to see if the cancer progresses is bound to cause prolonged periods of anxiety for many men; and therefore, a strong sense of commitment and mental stamina are demanded of those who choose to wait rather than be treated.

Early proponents of watchful waiting based their argument on Swedish data, which received a great deal of publicity back in the early 1990s. The Swedish researchers argued that there was no survival benefit for patients treated versus patients who were not treated. But if we look closely at those studies, it turns out that the patients were not just undergoing watchful waiting, because when the disease started to progress in men who had not been treated, they were subjected to endocrine therapies such as hormonal therapy or orchiectomy (castration). Therefore, the Swedish data did not provide an accurate picture of watchful waiting.

With regard to the Swedish data, it should be noted that orchiectomy or medical castration may in itself lead to increased risks of diabetes, high cholesterol, hypertension (HTN), and arteriosclerotic heart disease (ASHD), thus increasing the risk of stroke (cerebrovascular accident–CVA) and heart attack (myocardial infarction–MI). When all is said and done, patients in this Swedish study were determined to have died from causes other than prostate cancer, when in fact, it was the treatment of their prostate cancer with endocrine therapies that caused the early deaths.

It should also be noted that more recent research from Case Western University School of Medicine in Cleveland reported in November 2007 demonstrated that patients with localized prostate cancer cut their risk of dying of the disease in half when they have brachytherapy in conjunction with external radiation therapy compared to those men who do not get active treatment (watchful waiting) within six months of being diagnosed. Brachytherapy and external radiation therapy will be discussed at length in Chapter 6.

With regard to life expectancy, we often see reports in USA Today and other media sources that offer life tables that indicate American males are living an average of 75.4 years, but that's measured from birth. If you're already 70 years of age, you have a 14-year life expectancy. This was data reported in 2008 based on data from 2006. Patients are advised to check the table below to see what their life expectancy actually is. This is important if you opt for watchful waiting or expectant surveillance, because you may have the opportunity to get rid of your cancer now and put it behind you.

Many primary care doctors and many urologists are still in the old school, suggesting an average life expectancy for men of 75.4 years, while failing to take into account the increasing life expectancy for men who are 75 years and older. Some doctors have even suggested that older men should not be screened for prostate cancer. On August 8, 2008, the New York Times reported that the U.S. Preventative Services Task Force "recommended that doctors stop screening men ages 75 and older for prostate cancer because the search for the disease in this group was causing more harm than good." I challenge those guidelines. In my opinion, given recent trends in life expectancy for American males, a screening cutoff at age 75 is too early for many men who are otherwise in good health and can be effectively treated when diagnosed with the disease.

I believe older men should be evaluated on a case by case basis. The most recent SEER-Medicare data demonstrate a significant survival advantage for patients (ages 65 to 80) treated with radiation or surgery compared to patients who were not treated (Wong YN, et al, "Survival associated with treatment vs observation of localized prostate cancer in elderly men," JAMA. 2006 Dec 13;296(22):2683-93). Relatively noninvasive treatments, such as the most advanced radiation therapies (brachytherapy and/or IMRT), are often appropriate for older men, including those over 75, who are otherwise in good health—with less risk of surgical side effects that may reduce quality of life.

In addition, a recent study has shown that in the early 1990s as a result of PSA screening, the U.S. and U.K. had the same incidence of prostate cancer per capita; but since that time the U.S. has enjoyed more than a 4-fold decline in mortality compared to the U.K. And this was attributed directly to our TREATING elderly patients with definitive therapies vs watchful waiting, as is the method of choice in the U.K (Lancet Oncol. 2008 May;9(5):407-9).

According to the most recent actuarial data (National Vital Statistics Reports, June 11, 2008), a 75-year-old man can expect to live 10.9 years, and the trend is rising for all age groups. In the case of an 80-year-old whose general health is good and who has no other serious health conditions, he stands a good chance of living beyond 10 years and would be wise to consider treatment. A man's overall health should be considered as well as his age, since an 84 year old may actually be healthier than his 54 year old counterpart who smokes cigarettes, consumes excessive alcohol, etc. While many doctors continue to use 10 years life expectancy as a strict benchmark, when biopsy pathology and other lab tests identify aggressive, potentially life-threatening tumors, a 5-year cutoff may be indicated, and that would suggest screening is appropriate for many men over the age of 75, who can be effectively treated with radiation and/or hormonal therapy.

Projected Male Expectancy of Life: United States, 2006

AGE	AVG. LIFE EXPECTANCY
60	21.1 years
65	17.4
70	14
75	10.9
80	8.3
85	6.2
90	4.5

National Vital Statistics Reports, Vol 56, No. 16, 2008

CHAPTER TWO

THE DIAGNOSTIC TESTS
FOR PROSTATE CANCER

What is the Digital Rectal Exam (DRE)?

The digital rectal exam is the simplest way to detect physical abnormalities in the prostate gland that may suggest the presence of cancer. The DRE is also used to estimate the volume of the prostate and the extent of the cancer. The test is part of the physician's *work-up,* which involves a series of laboratory and radiographic tests that are used to determine how advanced the cancer is. The results of these tests will be evaluated to determine the *clinical stage* of the cancer, and they are also used to decide which type of treatment is most appropriate for your particular cancer.

To perform the rectal exam, the doctor feels the gland by placing a lubricated, gloved finger inside the rectum against the prostate (see Figure 4). When done properly, the test is not as discomforting as it might sound. Most cancers are located in the back of the prostate, and some of these cancers that have grown at the edge of the gland can be felt as a lump or hard nodule. Depending on the size, shape and location of the lump, it is sometimes possible to determine with a DRE if the cancer has spread beyond the prostate capsule. With the DRE, the doctor is able to evaluate some but not all portions of the gland's anatomy: portions of the right and lefts sides or *lobes;* the upper portion or *base* of the gland; the middle portion of the gland; and lower portion or *apex* (the latter two are most accurately palpated).

Unfortunately, the DRE is often not accurate. Many prostate cancers do not protrude against the back of the gland; they are not palpable and

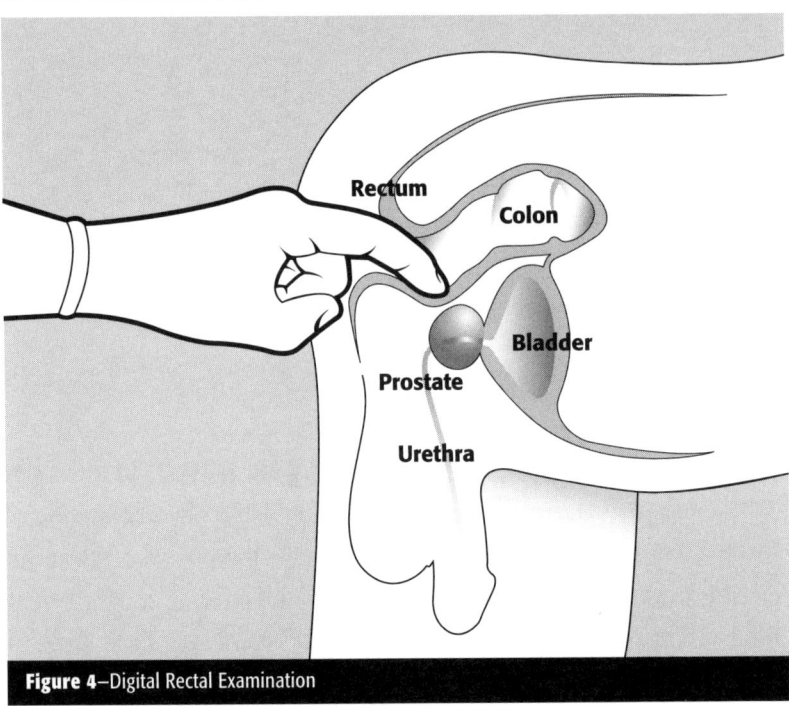

Figure 4–Digital Rectal Examination

cannot be detected with the DRE at all. A tumor at the front of the prostate cannot be felt through the rectum. In addition, the test is subjective and depends on the skill of the doctor, providing at best only an estimate of the extent of disease. Many surgical studies have shown that more than 50% of cancers that appear to be confined to the gland will later be found to have spread beyond the prostate capsule.

In my practice, I have found that performing the DRE with the patient in the dorso-lithotomy position (lying on back with legs raised) is much more accurate than the bend-over approach. With the former approach, the gland literally falls into the physician's finger, and the patient is less able to tighten the muscles around the gland.

What is the PSA test?

The PSA test was developed during the late 1970s by research scientists at Roswell Park Memorial Hospital in Buffalo, New York. The PSA is a blood test that measures the amount of *prostate specific antigen* (PSA) present in the body. Produced almost exclusively by the prostate gland, PSA is an enzyme, typically present in only minute quantities, secreted into the bloodstream from blood vessels inside the prostate.

PSA secretions originate from cells in the lining of the prostate gland. When prostate cancer is present, additional PSA is usually produced. This extra PSA can be detected and measured in the blood through a simple laboratory test, which can be ordered by any primary-care physician. Test results are usually available in 1-3 days or even longer depending on the assay used.

Because cancerous cells readily leak PSA into the surrounding body tissue, an elevated PSA is a possible indicator of the presence of prostate cancer. However, other conditions can also cause an elevated PSA. The most common is the enlargement of the prostate gland that occurs with BPH. Infections and traumas such as a biopsy or even an overly vigorous digital rectal exam can sometimes increase PSA levels. Ejaculation (orgasm) can elevate PSA for as long as 48 hours.

As a diagnostic tool, the PSA test has its limitations, and is usually combined with the DRE. Some men with seemingly normal PSA values turn out to have prostate cancer that may be detected with the DRE or one of the other diagnostic tests described in this chapter. A more aggressive cancer may be associated with a palpable tumor (at least a billion cells) found by DRE and a normal or even low PSA.

PSA—Typical ("Normal") range According to Age and Race

AGE	WHITE	ASIAN	AFRO-AMERICAN
40–49	0–2.5	0–2.0	0–2.0
50–59	0–3.5	0–3.0	0–2.0
60–69	0–4.5	0–4.0	0–4.5
70–79	0–6.5	0–5.0	0–5.5

How Are PSA Results Reported?

Standard PSA test results are reported in nanograms per milliliter (ng/ml), with a normal range of approximately 0-4 ng/ml. For the sake of simplicity, the units of measure will not be included in the remainder of this book when discussing PSA values. The normal range of PSA values must be adjusted slightly to account for differences in age and race (see box above). As men get older, the normal PSA range slowly increases. This normal range is generally lower for White males than for Asians and Afro-Americans.

Regardless of age and race factors, PSA levels greater than 10 are most often an accurate indicator of cancer. As many as 80 percent of men with this high a PSA reading (and a positive digital rectal exam) have been shown to have prostate cancer. Approximately 25 percent of those patients with a PSA between 4 and 10 turn out to have cancer, as confirmed by standard prostate biopsies. The accuracy of the PSA test is significantly improved when it is combined with the digital rectal exam. The PSA can detect twice as many cancers as the DRE alone; however, the DRE spots some cancers that may be missed by the PSA.

It should be stressed that the PSA test is not conclusive by itself in diagnosing prostate cancer. No treatment decision should ever be made on the basis of the PSA value by itself; however, an elevated PSA reading may suggest the need for further laboratory tests. A biopsy of the prostate gland is always necessary to confirm the presence of cancer.

Because the PSA test is not completely reliable as far as its predictive value, a patient with a high PSA level may not necessarily have cancer; and a patient with a very low PSA may not be cancer free. In fact, high grade, more aggressive cancers can lose their resemblance to prostate cells altogether and may not even produce PSA. The PSA provides only a statistical approximation, and there are often exceptions. PSA results are discussed in terms of probabilities—the likelihood of prostate cancer being present, and the likelihood that it may have spread beyond the prostate gland.

I'm often suspicious of any PSA greater than 2.5, especially with men who are 40 to 55 years old; however, I'm equally suspicious of a patient who has a normal PSA or even a low PSA, but an abnormal digital rectal examination. For example, if you have a man who has a prostate nodule and his PSA is 1.2, that's worth looking into with further testing. It may become even more concerning if he tells you that his father had prostate

What Factors Other Than Cancer Can Affect PSA Levels?

✔ Benign prostatic hyperplasia (BPH)

✔ Infection (prostatitis)

✔ Trauma such as biopsy or overly vigorous digital rectal examination (DRE)

✔ Ejaculation (up to a 40% elevation, returning to normal within 48 hours)

✔ Strenuous exercise involving the buttocks or perineum (such as bicycle riding)

✔ Medical procedures such as balloon dilation of the prostate, transrectal ultrasound-guided biopsy, and transurethral resection of the prostate (TURP)

✔ Medications such as finasteride (Proscar or Propecia) used to treat BPH can decrease PSA levels by as much as 50 percent.

✔ Various over the counter herbal mixtures marketed "for prostate health" may also affect PSA levels.

cancer or his brother had prostate cancer at an early age, or if he's an African-American. These are all considerations.

Once the presence of cancer is confirmed, the PSA results can be used to estimate the approximate size of the tumor, and the extent of the disease. The higher the PSA the more likely it is that the tumor is large and the cancer has extended beyond the prostate. Again, there are exceptions. Some patients with a high PSA may have small, curable cancers. Some men with a low PSA may have more advanced disease. Even with the exceptions and inaccuracies, the PSA test remains the most valuable tool available for diagnosing and monitoring prostate cancer.

The most important factor in deciding on treatment is whether or not the cancer has *metastasized*, that is, spread to parts of the body beyond the prostate. The higher the PSA value, the larger a tumor is likely to be, and the greater the likelihood that the cancer has spread outside the prostate capsule, unless the cancer is a non-PSA secreting tumor. Taken together, the PSA and DRE tests are very useful for detecting cancer, but they provide only rough estimates of how far the disease has actually progressed. As discussed later in this chapter and the next, more tests are necessary to determine the precise *stage* and *grade* of the disease. Staging and grading are standard systems for classifying the disease, that is, for evaluating the nature or grade of the malignancy, and the extent of the disease. All of this information is critical for deciding which treatment options are available for each patient.

Before having a biopsy, you should have your PSA tested several times at the same laboratory. There can be considerable variation with PSA test results depending on the lab and the particular test used. The FDA has approved a number of PSA tests, or assays, produced by various manufacturers; however, most of these tests have been approved only for PSA monitoring, not for diagnosis. Test results can vary by as much as 8 to 10 percent even when the test is done by the same laboratory. This variation is not considered significant, but it is important for patients to try to have their annual PSA test performed by the same lab each year, or at least to use the same FDA-approved brand of test.

Patients are advised to check with their local laboratory to find out what brand of PSA test is being used. Be sure the particular test at your lab has been FDA-approved for *both* diagnosis and monitoring of prostate cancer (some tests are approved only for monitoring). At our institution, we have established an advanced in-house blood lab that employs the third generation Immulite assay series produced by Diagnostic Products Corporation (DPC). These state of the art tests utilize a process known as *enzyme-amplified chemiluminescence,* which allows for highly sensitive PSA readings. One of the advantages of Immulite is greater precision as far as the number of decimal places reported (ie. to a level of less than 0.003 ng/ml). While not yet widely available, the Immulite assays are currently the most accurate PSA tests with FDA approval for diagnosis and for monitoring.

Why is There Controversy About the PSA Test?

Critics of PSA screening contend that the test detects many incidental, non-aggressive cancers that don't need to be diagnosed or treated because such cancers will never become life-threatening for the patient. The critics argue that many patients are being tested and treated unnecessarily. They also point out that studies have not yet proven definitively that any of the curative treatments for prostate cancer significantly improve survival. There are several ongoing studies to evaluate survival benefits of treatment. The SEER-Medicare Trial in the U.S. has demonstrated a statistically significant survival advantage for patients undergoing treatment, in contrast to older, flawed European studies. Even though the overall impact of treatment on survival is not yet conclusively established for each type of treatment, researchers have compiled extensive data (based on PSA monitoring and biopsy) to ascertain cure rates for each treatment modality.

Much of the controversy centers on the medical value of PSA screening and its cost-effectiveness. Critics are correct in pointing out that the PSA reports a significant percentage of "false positives," though at our institution we are finding less than about 10 percent of men with PSA readings over 10 do not have cancer. Some of these men will suffer the anxiety, inconvenience, and expense of further testing in order to rule out cancer. The fact remains that these tests can save many lives, and therefore, the cost and inconvenience appears to be justified. Although doctors have a difficult time distinguishing between cancers that are aggressive and those that are clinically insignificant, all prostate cancers are potentially life-threatening. Once prostate cancer is diagnosed, doctors have a responsibility to make their patients aware of their treatment options and the risks involved.

Critics argue that as many as 30 percent of men over the age of 50 have cancers that are insignificant, that will grow slowly and never cause any problem during their lifetimes. According to this argument, there is no point in diagnosing or treating these cancers. The fact is, however, that most prostate cancers diagnosed with PSA testing are clinically significant, and are potentially life-threatening, especially in light of the ever increasing life-expectancy of men discussed earlier. In a study conducted on men who were autopsied, no patient with a PSA greater than 4 had cancer that was clinically incidental. Moreover, in some men who appear to have incidental cancers, the disease will develop later, and they may eventually die of their cancer. The only way the large number of annual prostate cancer deaths is likely to be reduced is with early detection and treatment.

With that said, it should be emphasized that every man must make his own personal choice of whether to be tested for prostate cancer; and those patients who are diagnosed with the disease have the right to make the decision of whether or not to be treated. While there is no single treatment or set of answers for all patients, each man can make informed decisions about diagnosis and treatment.

The American Cancer Society (ACS) currently recommends that physicians offer the PSA test and DRE annually, beginning at age 50 for men who do not have any major medical problems and have a life expectancy of at least 10 more years. It is further recommended by the ACS that men at high risk, including African Americans and men with a family history of the disease, should begin testing at age 45. Men at even higher risk—for example, those with more than one close relative with prostate cancer diagnosed at an early age—could begin testing at age 40.

The ACS also encourages doctors to talk to men about the benefits and risks of testing. Men are encouraged to play an active role in making the choice about whether or not to be tested. Each man needs to be fully informed to make the decision that is right for him.

Based on recent studies, the American Urological Association (AUA) announced new PSA testing and screening guidelines in 2007, in the hope of reducing unnecessary biopsies and prostate surgeries. The new AUA guidelines will no longer rely on a single PSA reading. Rather, they suggest that doctors focus on changes in serum PSA levels over time (PSA velocity). They will also suggest that PSA testing start at age 40 to obtain a baseline, with the test repeated at 45 and 50, after which it should be given annually.

What is PSA Velocity?

PSA velocity refers to the rate of change of the PSA over time. The measurement of PSA velocity is known as PSAV or PSA slope. The assumption is that the annual rate of change of the PSA value for men with cancer is greater than for men without cancer, both those with normal prostate glands and those with BPH. A rise in the PSA of 0.75 or more in a year may be an indicator of cancer. A rise in the PSA less than 0.75 might indicate BPH, or could be a fluctuation attributed to a normal prostate.

Studies have shown that the use of PSA velocity can reduce the number of unnecessary biopsies. For patients with BPH, the number of biopsies may be reduced from 40 percent to 10 percent. PSA velocity can be especially telling for patients whose PSA is within the normal range but increasing rapidly. For example, a patient whose PSA rises from 1.3 to 2.3 to 3.7 over a period of two years might have a cancer detectable with a biopsy even before his PSA climbs above the normal limit of 4.0. This is where the benefit of early detection becomes most obvious, as the cancer can be caught when it is most treatable.

PSA velocity is also useful in diagnosing those patients whose PSA values are in the gray area between 4 and 10, and who have negative biopsies. For example, a patient with a 5.8 PSA value and negative biopsy might undergo another biopsy the following year if his PSA climbs significantly. An increase in PSA of less than 0.75 may rule out the need for another biopsy. The measurement of the PSA values over time greatly increases the ability of a doctor to make an accurate clinical diagnosis. For best results, the patient is usually advised to have his PSA tested at least three times over a period of two years.

While the PSA test can be very important, and may be the single most important marker to determine the likelihood of cancer being present, the PSA alone may not be as important as the PSA velocity. The history of the patient's PSA over time also enables us obtain the doubling time (PSADT) —the amount of time it takes for the PSA value to double—which can help us determine how rapidly the cancer is growing. A PSADT of less than 12 years and a PSA velocity greater than 0.75 indicate greater likelihood of malignancy.

What Are Free and Bound PSA?

Several other approaches for measuring PSA levels can allow us to make a more accurate diagnosis. Among these are free (or unbound) versus bound (or complexed) PSA. These terms refer to the fact that PSA appears in the bloodstream in two distinct molecular forms, either unattached to other substances (free), or combined with other protein molecules (bound). The percent-free PSA test measures how much PSA circulates free in the bloodstream compared to the total PSA level. The percentage of free PSA tends to be lower in men who have prostate cancer than in men who do not.

Some studies indicate that the amount of bound PSA in the blood is higher when cancer is present, while the amount of free PSA is higher in men with BPH. The percent-free PSA test is especially useful for diagnosing patients whose PSA falls into the gray area between 4 and 10, and even at lower levels between 2.5 and 4—when it is most difficult to distinguish cancer from benign enlargement of the prostate (BPH). By increasing the accuracy of PSA testing in this way, the number of unnecessary biopsies can be reduced. The percent-free PSA test may also be a valuable asset for monitoring patients after treatment. It should be noted that not every lab will perform a percent-free PSA test for patients with PSA values less than 4 or greater than 10.

What is PSA Density?

Another way we can sometimes distinguish between cancer and BPH is by measuring the PSA density, which is the PSA value divided by the volume of the prostate gland, as determined by transrectal ultrasound (discussed below). For a man with an enlarged prostate, the PSA value should not be greater than 15% of the weight of the prostate. Anything higher than that may be indicative of prostate cancer. The measurement of PSA density can help determine which men with slightly elevated PSA values should be subjected to biopsies to confirm or rule out the presence of cancer.

What is the PAP test?

At our institution, a PAP (Prostatic Acid Phosphatase) blood test is also routinely performed, as this test has been demonstrated by myself as well as others in the medical literature to be perhaps the single most adverse feature associated with prostate cancer. Before the advent of the PSA test, the PAP test was the only prostate tumor marker. In fact, doctors believed that the test was so accurate that if the patient had an elevated PAP, he should not undergo surgery because he would predictably have cancer beyond the prostate capsule, and therefore could not be cured by surgery.

After the advent of the PSA test and with the general excitement over the PSA marker, the PAP became less and less used. However, we never stopped using it and have even found that this test can be an independent prognosticator for treatment failure. In other words, in patients undergoing radiation therapy, we found that the PAP was as important as the PSA, and possibly more important for patients with advanced cancer, so we routinely employ it. Similar to radiation data, the PAP also carries tremendous statistical power for predicting whether or not a patient will relapse after surgery. Recent studies are finding that in patients with an elevated PAP, over 85% of those patients are going to fail after surgery. This should be no surprise in view of older pre-PSA surgical data. In contrast, however, while PAP is still an adverse prognosticator, at our institution, patients, despite having elevated PAPs, are being routinely treated using advanced radiation methods.

What is the PCA3Plus™ Test?

PCA3Plus™ is a urine-based genetic test for prostate cancer risk. This test detects PCA3, a specific gene that is highly expressed in prostate cancer. In fact, no other human tissues express PCA3.

This genetic test is the second generation of another highly successful test known as uPM3™. PCA3Plus™ tests for prostate cancer cells that are shed into the urine (following a digital rectal exam). The urine sample is sent to Bostwick Laboratories, Inc. to be tested for genetic expression of the PCA3 gene. If the sample tests positive for PCA3, then the patient has a very high likelihood of having prostate cancer. PCA3Plus™, when validated by Bostwick Laboratories predicts prostate cancer with a sensitivity of 95.7%.

PCA3Plus™ has not yet been approved by the FDA, and is based upon reagents which are manufactured by Gen-Probe (San Diego, California). PCA3PlusTM is a trademark of Bostwick Laboratories, Inc, with corporate headquarters in Glen Allen, Virginia. uPM3™ is a trademark of Diagno-Cure (Quebec City, Quebec, Canada).

One advantage of the PCA3Plus™ genetic test is that it can help reduce the number of prostate biopsies based on PSA and DRE tests (see below,

"What is a Prostate Biopsy?). According to researchers at the Johns Hopkins University School of Medicine, due to elevated PSA levels, approximately 1.6 million men undergo prostatic biopsies in the U.S. annually, and roughly 80% of these men end up having negative results.

As doctors add to their arsenal of diagnostic work-up tests, early detection of the disease becomes more accurate and reliable. Doctors at Johns Hopkins are working with another serum marker known as Early Prostate Cancer Antigen-2 (EPCA-2) which may one day further reduce the number of unnecessary prostate biopsies (Leman ES, et al, EPCA-2: "A highly specific serum marker for prostate cancer," *Urology,* 2007 Apr; 69(4):714-20).

What is a Prostate Biopsy?

A prostate biopsy is a procedure by which samples of tissue are removed from suspicious areas of the prostate gland for microscopic examination by a pathologist. A biopsy is absolutely necessary to confirm the presence of cancer and should be undertaken prior to any treatment of the disease. The biopsy may also provide us with a wealth of information about the specific characteristics of the cancer.

When performing a biopsy, the doctor will use an imaging technique called transrectal ultrasound (TRUS) for guidance in order to insert a narrow needle through the wall of the rectum into the prostate gland. A grayscale ultrasound is most commonly used. Doctors can also perform the biopsy through the perineum, the area between the rectum and scrotum. This is known as a "transperineal biopsy." The needle removes a tiny core of tissue (usually measuring about 1/2-inch by 1/16-inch) that is sent to the laboratory to see if cancer is present. Although the procedure may sound painful, a biopsy usually causes little discomfort because an instrument called a biopsy gun inserts and removes the needle in a fraction of a second. In addition, a local or regional anesthetic should be used to numb the area. The procedure can be performed in the doctor's office and usually takes only about 15 minutes. In contrast, transperineal biopsies are typically performed in a hospital setting during a very short "one day procedure admission."

The prostate biopsy has traditionally involved obtaining at least six core samples of tissue. This procedure, known as the sextant biopsy, draws tissue from the base, mid-gland and apex for a total of six core samples. Recent studies have shown that increasing the number of samples can significantly increase the detection of malignancy. The number of biopsy samples taken now typically ranges from 6 to 18 or more, with the standard being 12. The 5-region biopsy approach obtains additional samples from the mid-gland tissue and the lateral zones or lobes on each side of the gland. When a very large number of samples are obtained, this approach is called "saturation biopsy" and is best performed using the transperineal method.

Your biopsy report should indicate how many tissue samples were taken from specific areas of the prostate, and how many specimens showed cancer. The report should also indicate what percentage of each core contained cancer and how many specimens showed solid cores. If each core is solid, then the tumor is likely to be large. If the cores are small and scattered, the needle probably passed through small tumors. More than 50% cancer in any one core and/or multiple positive cores would suggest a larger tumor. When more than half of a prostate lobe is involved, the outlook is less optimistic because larger tumors have a less favorable prognosis. Your doctor will use all of this information about the size and extent of your cancer, along with the results of the rest of the work-up tests, to develop a strategy for treating the disease. It should be noted that because of the gray-scale ultrasound and its inability to "see" or accurately locate the cancer, a biopsy specimen obtained this way is only as good as the region or tumor located.

Recent studies have shown that biopsies guided by the color-flow Doppler ultrasound imaging technique (see discussion below) have the advantage of showing the optimal sites from which to secure tissue samples. Once the initial diagnosis has been established, I typically request that the specimen slides be reviewed by a pathologist who specializes in prostate pathology. Specialists in evaluating prostate biopsy specimens are available at a number of labs and major medical centers. Samples can be sent to these specialists for "second opinions," as the pathological interpretation can vary. There is an "art" to interpreting the slides, and it is that interpretation that your doctor will use in determining how to best treat the disease.

With respect to saturation biopsies, in my practice, I perform them for both practical and theoretical reasons. The procedure is commonly re-

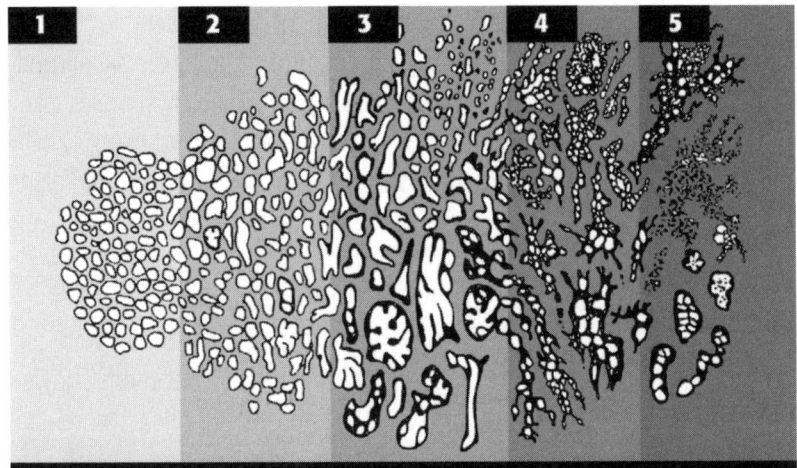

Figure 5—A simplified drawing of the Gleason grading system, showing the five distinct grades of cancerous tissue, as seen under low magnification. The two most common cell patterns seen in the tissue sample are added together to arrive at a Gleason score.

ferred to as "template-guided transperineal 3-dimensional mapping (3-DMP)." This technique is virtually the same as performing brachytherapy (see Chapter 6, "What is Brachytherapy?") from the standpoint of patient positioning (dorso-lithotomy), using a regional anesthetic, and using the brachytherapy template grid. The only real difference is that seeds are not deposited but rather tissue is extracted using a biopsy gun.

This approach avoids some of the limitations associated with the standard transrectal approach. These include the ability to better access and sample the apical prostate (lowest portion), anterior prostate (transitional zone) and the most postero-lateral (left and right) aspects of the gland, all of which can be challenging and sometimes simply not possible with the standard method (especially in larger glands).

The risk of infection is less with the 3-DMP approach as is the degree of rectal bleeding, since the "contaminated" rectal wall is not pierced, while only a betadine cleansed "sterile" perineum is pierced using the 3-DMP method. Its only drawback is that it is much more costly. At our institution, we have a policy to perform the 3-DMP method only as a follow-up approach to one or two negative sets of standard in-office Color Flow Doppler biopsies OR in cases where it is clear that the abnormal area(s) of color flow perfusion is(are) outside of where we feel we can reach with the biopsy gun using the standard technique. One additional advantage to the 3-DMP method is that it may better determine which cases can be theoretically managed with "watchful waiting" or "expectant management," that is, patients having "insignificant cancer," since the likelihood of "undersampling of the disease" is very small (*J Urol* 2002,167:1231-1234).

What is the Gleason Score?

Under the microscope, prostate cancer cells exhibit a particular range of aggressiveness, from slow-growing to fast-growing, and they are ranked accordingly. The ranking used to identify how aggressive or abnormal a cancer appears is called the Gleason scale. The scale essentially runs from 2 to 10, with the least aggressive tumors at the low end and the fastest growing, more aggressive tumors at the high end of the scale.

Slow-growing tumors appear similar to normal tissue and are called "well-differentiated." Fast-growing cancers appear abnormal and are called "poorly differentiated." Between the two extremes are cancers which are classified as moderately differentiated." The Gleason system defines five glandular patterns of cancerous cell tissue, from completely differentiated to completely undifferentiated. Tumors often possess more than one cellular pattern, and therefore, both primary and secondary patterns are graded. The two grades are combined to get the actual Gleason score, ranging from 2 (1 + 1) to 10 (5 + 5), with most cancers falling somewhere in between (See Figure 5).

The higher the Gleason score, the more likely it is that the cancer is more aggressive and has already spread beyond the prostate capsule or metastasized to other parts of the body. Unfortunately, like the PSA scale, the Gleason scale provides only an approximation of how aggressive a cancer is and how likely it is that the cancer has spread. One part of the prostate gland may appear to be more aggressive or abnormal than other parts, and there is some element of chance as to where exactly the needle obtains each specimen.

The imprecision of Gleason scoring creates exceptions when interpreting the numbers. Some men with high Gleason scores may have small, curable cancers, while other men with lower numbers may have cancers that are more advanced. Nevertheless, the Gleason score is fairly accurate in predicting how aggressive the cancer is and how rapidly it will spread. However, it should be noted again that there are limitations to the biopsy that utilizes gray-scale ultrasound for guidance, and the Gleason score is only a reflection of that portion of the tumor which the physician biopsies. Using the gray-scale machine, a non-aggressive cancer may be biopsied while a more aggressive cancer is missed.

What is Transrectal Ultrasound (TRUS)?

Technically referred to a *transrectal ultrasonography*, this is a technique that projects sound waves off the prostate and surrounding organs to create an image. The sound waves are generated by a probe placed inside the rectum. Transrectal ultrasound imaging can in many cases accurately identify the local spread of cancer through the prostate capsule. In some cases, however, areas of cancer growth through the prostatic capsule may be too small to be visible, especially when using gray-scale ultrasound. As mentioned, ultrasound is often used to guide the biopsy needle to suspicious sites in the prostate. The technique is also used for real time guidance in conjunction with seed implants, external radiation therapy, and other treatments.

At our institution, color-flow Doppler ultrasound is utilized since it provides enhanced visualization and greater definition compared to the conventional gray-scale technique. While there is an art to interpreting color-flow Doppler images, tumors tend to demonstrate increased blood perfusion or *hypervascularity* as findings consistent with malignancy. Tumors are growing faster than normal prostate cells and require more blood to nurture their growth. Tumors therefore tend to create blood vessels around them as they grow, and these abnormal vascular patters can be identified by color-flow Doppler ultrasound. A conventional TRUS typically shows what are called *hypoechogenic* areas, which are darker shades of gray. A color-flow Doppler ultrasound will also show the same image, but it provides additional insight into how much perfusion of blood is going into the region, and can reveal whether just one prostate nodule is involved or if there is more cancer dispersed throughout the gland.

What are CT Scans and Fused Imaging Modalities?

The CT scan (also called CAT scan) uses *computer tomography* to produce a 3-dimensional image of the prostate and surrounding organs. CT scans rely on computer-reconstructed x-rays to give a cross-sectional view of the body. A CT scan through the pelvis reveals the outline of the prostate.

CT scans can identify prostate enlargement and show the size and shape of the gland, but it is not as effective for assessing the extent of cancer or visualizing cancer within the gland itself. While CT scans provide less defined images of the outer prostatic contour and internal architecture, CT images do accurately delineate the spatial relationship between the prostate, rectum and pubic bones. More contemporary spiral or helical CT scans provide greater resolution while taking less time to acquire the information, and thus, far less radiation exposure. The latest CT software enables full 3-dimensional resolution.

The arm of the CT scanner directs pinpoint-thin x-ray beams through the portions of the body under examination as it rapidly passes over the patient. Each pass of the CT scanner provides a cross-section of the body's internal structures, and as many as eight scans per centimeter are taken.

The data is fed into a computer, which converts the information into a three-dimensional image. The image gives a more precise and accurate picture of the internal organs than the flat view provided by a conventional x-ray, which superimposes overlapping organs and can only dimly represent the soft tissues of the body.

Today the CT scan is often combined or fused with other sophisticated imaging and diagnostic modalities, such as the MRI scan, PET scan, ProstaScint® and Combidex® tests (see also below, "What is a ProstaScint® Scan?"). These fused imaging modalities represent the state of the art and have greatly enhanced our ability to diagnose and treat the disease.

What is an Endorectal MRI?

MRI refers to *magnetic resonance imaging,* a state of the art technique that generates a magnetic field, which harmlessly reacts with the tissues of the body to produce a distinct and complex image of internal organs. The endorectal MRI utilizes a rectal probe to provide sharper images and is especially useful in detecting capsular penetration. The MRI is primarily used in staging biopsy-proven prostate cancer. This imaging technique is more accurate than CT scans or standard gray-scale ultrasound for detecting cancer that has penetrated the prostate capsule. However, approximately 30% of patients who do not show capsular penetration with MRI may still have some penetration that is too small to be detected.

While its availability is limited in the U.S., magnetic resonance spectroscopic imaging (MRSI) is the most discriminating test in terms of both the internal architecture of the prostate gland and determining whether or not the cancer has spread beyond the prostate capsule, which is termed *extracapsular extension* (ECE). With its high degree of detail, the endorectal MRI can show whether or not there is rectal or seminal vesicle involvement. Bladder invasion can also be detected by an endorectal MRI, while it's not commonly seen with a CT scan or with a conventional gray-scale ultrasound study.

The endorectal MRI is much like an ultrasound probe in that it is placed in the rectum and allows you to image the prostate very closely. It's as detailed a test as you can get in terms of looking at the capsule of the prostate and determining whether or not there is cancer that has extended outside of the prostate capsule.

There is a current debate over whether a more powerful magnet (3.0 Tesla versus 1.5 Tesla) may obviate the need for the endorectal probe. In addition, the "dynamic" MRI is challenging the spectroscopic MRI as the true gold standard. Approximately 90% of our patients undergo a dynamic or spectroscopic MRI with or without the endorectal coil. The choice of dynamic versus spectroscopic with or without endorectal coil is made on a case by case basis. The only reason a patient wouldn't have an MRI is if his insurance company would not pay for it and the patient can't afford the test, as it is expensive. The cost of a diagnostic pelvic MRI is at least two to three times higher than the cost for a TRUS or CT scan.

What is a Bone Scan?

A bone scan is an imaging technique used to detect bone metastases, which appear as "hot spots" on film. It is far more sensitive than conventional x-rays. The bone scan procedure is performed by injecting a small amount of radioactive dye called *technetium* into the patient's bloodstream. A special camera is then used to photograph the skeleton, and any irritation of the bone will show up as a spot on the image.

If a patient's PSA is high, greater than 10, or if the Gleason score is greater than or equal to 7, then I usually recommend a bone scan. Similarly, a bone scan is also recommended if a patient has a low PSA yet palpable disease and/or a Gleason score suggesting aggressive disease. A spot on a bone scan may be caused by cancer that has metastasized, or by arthritis and other causes. When an abnormality shows up on a bone scan, further tests such as traditional x-rays, CT or MRI may be used to determine if the cause is cancer. It is important to establish a baseline to differentiate between cancer and other abnormalities.

Most of our patients undergo an 18F-FDG Fluoride PET / CT Fusion study, which has a predictive accuracy of 98%. This avoids the false positive and false negative rates which may be associated with bone scans (as a result of the 18F tumor-imaging agent). Meanwhile, the FDG portion of this test may pick up Gleason 8 to 10 prostate cancers in the lymph nodes, as well as other cancers which may as yet not have been detected in the body (e.g. lung cancers, gastrointestinal malignancies, head and neck cancers, and lymphomas).

What is a ProstaScint® Scan?

ProstaScint® is a staging test that utilizes a radioactive isotope, which is attached to a *monoclonal antibody* (mAb), which targets a specific cancer protein know as *prostate specific membrane antigen* (PSMA). After this combined isotope-mAb is injected into the bloodstream, it will track down that particular cancer protein and then attaches to it. This is an imaging test rather than a blood test *per se.* Three to four days after being injected, a patient is scanned with a special camera that picks up the radiation emitted by the isotope and locates the cancer.

If a patient's PSA is very high, for example, in excess of 20, or if there are other additional factors like a Gleason score of 8 or higher, or an elevated PAP, then a patient should probably undergo a ProstaScint® study. I use this test for patients whom I suspect are at a high risk for having cancer which has gone beyond the prostate gland. The ProstaScint® studies may lend some important information for these patients because it tells us a great deal about soft tissue. If there is lymph node involvement, a Prosta-Scint® scan may show the cancer going very accurately and methodically from the prostate gland up to the internal iliac or lymph node chain, or to known sites or banks where prostate cancer commonly goes.

As yet, not many institutions use the ProstaScint® scan although its availability is growing and it is FDA approved. It can be a revealing test, but again, it should be limited to patients having more aggressive cancer. I wouldn't put everyone through it since it's associated with false positives and it's expensive. One of its advantages, however, is that while other tests may be affected by a patient being on hormones, the ProstaScint® scan should still be predictably effective because it's looking for PSMA rather than PSA. Compared to PSA, only relatively small amounts of PSMA are detectable in the bloodstream of prostate cancer patients.

Fusing the ProstaScint® with a helical CT study or MRI significantly improves the predictive accuracy of the ProstaScint® test (fewer false positives and negatives). In patients with Gleason 8 to 10 tumors, a Prosta-Scint®/ CT / PET Fusion may be dictated. Fusion studies are relatively new and are only as good as the technologist performing it and the radiologist interpreting it. Like everything else in this field, it pays to search out experienced practitioners who deal with a large case load.

What is a Lymphadenectomy?

Lymphadenectomy, or removal of lymph nodes, is a surgical procedure which looks at the lymph node-bearing sites that prostate cancer can drain to. As with any part of the body when cancer is present, there is always a station of lymph nodes where cancer can collect or accumulate. The lymph nodes are scavengers of abnormal things in the body. The prostate gland has its own stations of lymph nodes, the primary ones being the obturator lymph nodes and the internal iliac lymph nodes. These reside in the pelvis. Once the lymph nodes collect cancer, they often disperse the cancer into the blood stream.

My personal opinion is that an exploratory lymphadenectomy is a far more rigorous and invasive procedure than a relatively non-invasive primary treatment such as a seed implant. Urologists rarely do formal lymphadenectomies, probably because it is a morbid procedure in and of itself. I generally favor giving the patient the benefit of the doubt by doing an implant, barring obvious metastases to the lymph nodes or obvious lymph node spread, as determined by radiographic studies. Given the fact that we are demonstrating successful treatment results even in patients who have lymph node spread, by using other combined treatment methods such as hormonal therapies followed by sophisticated radiation techniques, lymphadendectomies would add little but morbidity to the picture.

Laparoscopic lymph node dissection is a less invasive procedure than lymphadenectomy and may be more attractive, but the laparascopic procedure is also less accurate. Nonetheless, if a ProstaScint® Fusion study is highly suggestive of lymph node involvement, directed laparascopic lymph node sampling may be useful. The use of "sentinel" lymph node tracking is also gaining increasing popularity.

What is Ploidy Analysis?

Another test sometimes performed by the pathologist utilizes a hi-tech examination called *flow cytometry* to analyze the nuclear DNA content, or *DNA Ploidy*, of cancer cells. Samples for analysis may be obtained from biopsy or operating tissue. The genetic information derived from this test allows cancer cells to be classified as "diploid," "tetraploid," or "aneuploid."

Aneuploid cancers generally have a less favorable prognosis than diploid cancers, and if left untreated are more likely to progress rapidly. Diploid cancers have a more favorable prognosis than either aneuploid or tetraploid. Why ploidies differ and why some indicate a more aggressive cancer than others remains the subject of continuing research.

While this method of analysis is very sensitive, the predictive value of flow cytometry is not definitive, and the test is not reliable enough to be used by itself as a diagnostic tool. As far as determining the aggressiveness of the tumor, ploidy can be enhanced when combined with the patient's PSA and Gleason score. It is a subject of debate whether the data on ploidy is solid enough to be used as a basis for treatment decisions. Most physicians do not rely on this form of testing. When ploidy is used, it is most often called for when the patient's Gleason score is greater than or equal to 7. Some studies have suggested that if the PSA is greater than or equal to 15, and if the ploidy is aneuploid, then the likelihood is that the cancer will already have metastasized to the lymph nodes or beyond.

What Other Tests are Commonly Used?

Depending on the specifics of the case, a number of other tests may be utilized and are commonly used in my practice. Their names may sound like alphabet soup, but they are all useful in determining the extent and aggressiveness of the cancer. Don't be put off by the medical terminology. Patients should not be reluctant to discuss with their doctors the purpose of each of these laboratory tests as they relate to their own individual cases.

Some of these tests, or *markers,* may be used to identify mutant tumor populations, or aggressive tumors in patients without elevated PSAs. Markers of this type include NSE (Neuron Specific Enolase), CGA (Chromagranin A), and CEA (Carcinoembryonic Antigen). A number of other lab tests help to determine whether or not some form of hormonal therapy may be indicated either in the short term or at a later date. These tests include those that measure levels of Testosterone (total and bio-available), DHT (dihydrotestosterone), DHEA-S (dehyrdoepiandrosterone sulphate), Estradiol, Prolactin, LH (Luteinizing Hormone) and Androstenedione.

Other evaluative procedures, such as Urine Pyrilinks-D™ (Dpd), N-telopeptide (serum or urine), and Bone Specific Alkaline Phosphatase, are often used in addition to a Bone Mineral Density (BMD) test to establish a baseline for bone integrity. This is especially important for patients undergoing hormonal therapy, which can cause bone loss or resorption. With regard to the BMD test, in my practice, a quantitative computerized tomography (QCT) scan is preferred over the Dual Energy X-ray Absorptiometry (DEXA) scan, as the QCT provides more accurate results. Additional tests such as a urine cytology study and NMP-22 bladder cancer marker may be used to evaluate for other malignancies. Tests such as IGF-1 and IL-6 may be included in a systemic evaluation.

There are other areas within the pathology itself which we may want to examine. Whether or not a cancer has attached itself to a nerve *(perineural invasion or PNI)* is important because we know that a nerve typically tracks throughout the gland and outside of the gland, and that it can act as something of a conduit for the cancer. Perineural invasion essentially allows the cancer to get a free ride outside the prostate gland proper. When pathological examination indicates extensive PNI, there is an enormous likelihood of extra-prostatic extension, such as capsular penetration and/or seminal vesicle involvement. In addition, genetic markers like bcl2, p27, p53, and MIB-1 may help to determine the aggressiveness of tumors. These markers are obtained from immuno-histochemical stains from the initial tumor block (biopsied tissue).

CHAPTER THREE

CONSIDERATIONS PRIOR TO TREATMENT

How Much Time is There to Make a Decision About Treatment?

If you are a newly diagnosed patient, you should not be concerned that the several weeks which may be required for testing and consultations with your doctor will give the cancer time to grow and spread. In most cases, prostate cancer is slow to progress, as indicated by the slow rise of PSA values over time. In fact, by the time most men are diagnosed, they have already had the disease for several years. Judging by the slow rise of PSA levels, a newly diagnosed patient should be able to safely devote a month or so to becoming informed about the disease and learning about his treatment options. It is extremely unlikely that investing that amount of time will decrease the likelihood of a man being cured.

There may be rare exceptions to such a time frame when a patient's PSA doubling time is only 3 to 6 months, with a PSA of greater than 20 and a Gleason score of 8 to 10. With such a rapidly growing, aggressive cancer, the situation may warrant more expeditious research to determine the best treatment option, which should be undertaken without lengthy delays.

What is the Difference Between Early Stage and Metastatic Disease?

Deciding which treatments are appropriate in large part depends on the stage or extent of the cancer as indicated by the results of the work-up tests. The evaluation of stage is based on the doctor's interpretation of the test results. Different types of treatment are available as options for each patient depending on whether the cancer is locally confined to the prostate gland and nearby tissues, or whether the cancer has metastasized to distant parts of the body.

Early stage prostate cancer refers to small and medium size tumors that are most likely to be totally confined within the prostate. This stage is sometimes called *organ-confined disease* (OCD). *Locally advanced disease* is defined as cancer that has spread beyond the confines of the prostate proper (e.g. a bulky tumor extending into the periprostatic tissue or invading the seminal vesicles, bladder or rectum. The term *metastatic disease* indicates that the cancer has spread to the regional lymph nodes or distant sites such as bone, lungs or liver.

In the case of metastatic disease, microscopic clumps of cancer cells break away from the original tumor and travel via the bloodstream or lymph system to another location of the body, where new tumors start to grow. These metastatic tumors, wherever they have formed, are made of the same kind of cells as the original tumor. Prostate cancer that has spread to the bones does not become bone cancer. It is prostate cancer outside the prostate, and needs to be treated accordingly.

As the cancerous growth expands, it presses on surrounding tissues and replaces healthy cells at the perimeter of the mass. As it grows in size, symptoms of the disease will eventually start to appear. These vary depending on the site and nature of the cancer. Metastatic disease will typically extend to the regional lymph nodes, and then to the bones of the hip or lower back. While the likelihood of cure is very small, advanced disease can be treated in order to slow the progression of the cancer and to relieve symptoms. We have had considerable success treating patients with minimal to modest pelvic lymph node involvement when compared to those having extensive lymph node metastases.

What are the Stages of Prostate Cancer?

A staging system is a standardized way to classify the extent to which the disease has spread. Decades of studies have led to the classification of prostate cancer into essentially four distinct stages. These were initially identified as A, B, C, and D in the Whitmore-Jewett system, which dates from 1956. There are sub-stages for each stage of prostate cancer as well. The stage is based on factors such as the size or volume of disease, Gleason grade, and spread of disease beyond the prostate or to other sites in the body, such as the seminal vesicles, pelvic lymph nodes, or more distant sites such as lungs or bones. Accurate staging of the disease is crucial to developing an appropriate treatment plan.

Since 1992, most physicians have switched over to a newer staging system known as TNM (tumor, nodes, metastases) that describes the extent of the primary tumor (in stages ranging from T1 through T4), whether the cancer has invaded the regional lymph nodes (N stage), and whether the cancer has metastasized (M stage). The TNM system roughly parallels the A to D classification system, but the TNM system subdivides each stage in more detail. The TNM system has been revised over the years, and the most recent is that which appears in the 2002 staging manual of the American Joint Committee on Cancer (AJCC).

The stages are classified as follows:

T Stages: There are two types of T classifications. The *clinical stage* is an assessment made on the basis of clinical tests performed without direct examination of the tumor or cancer cells. The classifications described in this section are primarily based on clinical evaluation. Although the tests used in staging are always undergoing improvement, clinical staging is a subjective process, and therefore, not foolproof. Staging tests provide valuable information to the physician, but unavoidable errors in assessing the stage still do occur. The *pathological stage* provides more precise and verifiable data on the extent of the disease. It is accomplished by means of biopsy and surgical exploration.

Stage T1 (also known as Stage A): These are cancers confined to the prostate that cannot be felt during rectal examination and produce no symptoms. These tumors usually cannot be seen with ultrasound or other imaging techniques. Stage T1 tumors are often found by accident during routine examination of tissue removed during surgery for benign prostatic hypertrophy (BPH). As many as 10% of men who undergo transurethral resection of the prostate (TURP) for BPH are discovered to have unsuspected prostate cancer. This stage is further divided into three sub-stages.

Stage T1a: Although there is some variance in definitions of this sub-stage, it typically describes a "focalized tumor" (spherical and possessing a distinct boundary between the tumor and surrounding tissue) that comprises 5% or less of the surgical specimen.

Stage T1b: Typically a "diffuse tumor" that comprises over 5% of the removed specimen of prostate tissue. Note that T1a and T1b are stages which are most often detected incidentally following a TURP.

Stage T1c: The tumor is not palpable and usually identified by biopsy performed after determination of an elevated PSA.

Stage T2 (also know as Stage B): The tumor can be felt by rectal examination, but is still confined to the prostate gland.

Stage T2a: The tumor is palpable and involves less than one half of one side or lobe of the prostate.

Stage T2b: The cancer is palpable and involves more than one half of one lobe but not both lobes of the prostate gland.

Stage T2c: The cancer is palpable and involves both lobes.

Stage T3 and T4 (also known as Stage C): These are tumors that have extended through the prostatic capsule (extracapsular extension), and are no longer confined to the prostate. Stage T3 and T4 cancers often involve most or all of the prostate gland, and the entire prostate may feel hard upon rectal examination.

Stage T3a: The tumor has extended through the prostatic capsule on one side or two sides (unilateral or bilateral extracapsular extension).

Stage T3b: The cancer has spread to the seminal vesicles. Often symptoms of the disease will begin to appear at this stage, such as difficulty urinating.

Stage T4: The tumor has invaded structures adjacent to the prostate other than the seminal vesicles, most commonly the rectum and/or bladder.

Stage T4a: The tumor has invaded the bladder neck, rectum or external sphincter.

Stage T4b: The tumor has invaded the levator muscles and/or is fixed to the pelvic wall.

N Stages: These stages describe regional lymph node involvement.

Stage NX: Indicates the regional lymph nodes have not been assessed.

Stage N0: Indicates the cancer has not spread to the lymph nodes.

Stage N1 (also known as Stage D1): The cancer has spread beyond the prostate and invaded a single regional lymph node, 2 cm. or smaller.

Stage N2: Cancer has spread to one or more regional lymph nodes, 2 cm. or larger, but not larger than 5 cm. in greatest diameter.

Stage N3: Cancer has spread to a regional lymph node and is larger than 5 cm in greatest diameter.

M Stages: These stages describe distant metastasis.

MX: Indicates distant metastasis cannot be assessed.

M0: Indicates there is no distant metastasis.

M1 (also known as Stage D2): The cancer has spread to distant sites in the body. Metastatic disease will often spread to nearby bones, but may also involve the liver, lungs or other tissues.

M1a: Indicates non-regional lymph node involvement.

M1b: Indicates cancer that has spread to the bones.

M1c: Indicates cancer that has spread to other sites with or without bone disease.

As indicated by biopsy and surgical exploration, pathological stages include the following:

pT2: Organ confined

    pT2a: Unilateral

    pT2b: Bilateral

pT3: Extraprostatic extension

    pT3a: Extraprostatic extension

    pT3b: Seminal vesicle invasion

pT4: Invasion of bladder, rectum

As discussed in the previous chapter, there are a wide variety of staging tests, each possessing unique capabilities and serving a specific function in the staging process. Some tests are used to visualize the internal structures of the body, such as the CT scan, ultrasound (especially 3-D color-flow Doppler TRUS), endorectal MRI (magnetic resonance imaging,) or 3D-MRSI (three dimensional, magnetic resonance spectrographic imaging). These techniques allow doctors to improve their assessment of cancer location and extent within the prostate.

Other tests are used to identify the presence of cancer in various parts of the body, such as the chest x-ray or bone scan. Blood tests such as the PSA and PAP may be used to give a general indication of the extent and aggressiveness of the disease. These tests can be used for preliminary staging and for subsequent staging to track changes in a patient's illness or evaluate the effectiveness of treatment.

What Factors Determine Low, Intermediate and High Risk Patients?

With respect to risk assessment definitions of prostate cancer, many doctors use the American Joint Committee on Cancer (AJCC) 2002 risk stratification guidelines. These guidelines define low risk patients as those having a serum PSA less than 10, a Gleason score less than or equal to 6, and the stage less than or equal to T2b. In addition, for low risk patients, many doctors also note that the endorectal MRI or spectroscopic MRI and color-flow Doppler ultrasound should not demonstrate more extensive tumor than was anticipated. According to the AJCC 2002 guidelines, with inter-mediate risk, the PSA is greater than or equal to 10, the Gleason is greater than or equal to 7, and the stage is greater than or equal to T2c. Patients in the high risk group have at least two of those factors.

Risk Categorization Definitions (per 2002 AJCC)					
RISK	PSA		GLEASON		STAGE
LOW	<10		≤6		≤T2b
INTERMEDIATE	≥10	or	≥7	or	≥T2c
HIGH At least 2 of these factors	≥10		≥7		≥T2c

Another set of risk stratification guidelines is identified by the National Comprehensive Cancer Network Staging Guidelines). The two guidelines are very similar—patients who have higher volume and higher grade dis-ease are placed in the high risk group.

National Comprehensive Cancer Network Staging Guidelines			
RISK	PSA	GLEASON	STAGE
LOW	<10	≤6	≤T2a
INTERMEDIATE	10–20	=7	T2b–T2c
HIGH	>20	≥8	≥T3

As many doctors treat both intermediate and high risk patients similarly, these patients are routinely grouped together. They may have a clinical stage tumor which is greater than or equal to T2B, a PSA greater than 10, Gleason score greater than or equal to 7 and/or an elevated PAP. Intermedi-ate risk patients typically have only one of these risk factors, while high risk patients possess two or more. If a PSA is extremely high or if a PAP is very high, it often means that the cancer has left the prostate gland, although it may not mean that it has spread widely into the bloodstream, but may be suggestive of cancer spreading to tissues around the prostate and/or the lymph nodes (locally advanced disease). These patients are still curable, although that is very unlikely with surgery.

There are other tests and factors that are also taken into account when assessing risk. Evidence of perineural invasion and/or ploidy status (for example, an aneuploid tumor) may predict a less favorable prognosis, and as such, patients having these features are most commonly treated in the intermediate to high-risk category. The same applies to other adverse indicators such as the suppressor gene P27 and the monoclonal antibody MIB1. Genes that relate to tumor growth (oncogenes) such as bcl-2 and growth factors obtained in serum analysis such as TGF beta-1 may also portend more aggressive, higher risk cancers. While these clinical, laboratory, pathology and radiology findings may sound like complicated medical jargon, they are actually crucial pieces of information that your doctor can use to create a profile of the cancer that will help you in making the difficult decisions about treatment.

As indicated previously, a patient's treatment options in large part depend on exactly how far the cancer has spread. Accurate staging allows us to determine the probability of whether or not the cancer has escaped the prostate capsule. There are a number of powerful tools that enable us to predict which patients—those having certain clinical stages, PSA levels and Gleason scores—may harbor extracapsular extension (cancer that has escaped the prostate capsule) as well as lymph node involvement. These tools are statistical approaches to risk assessment that allow doctors and patients to know what to expect given their individual test results. The statistical calculations are based on data found in peer-reviewed medical literature that relate various disease indices (such as stage, PSA and Gleason scores) to outcomes reported with each type of treatment.

One of the original risk assessment tools is called the Partin Tables, named after its originator, Dr. Alan Partin, of Johns Hopkins University. The Partin Tables are based on problem-solving "algorithm" procedures, a series of complex analyses and formulas for assessing a patient's risk. Using this statistical approach, patients are able to plug their own data into formulas that reveal the probability of the cancer being confined to the prostate. The tables also predict the likelihood of extracapsular penetration, as well as lymph node and seminal vesicle involvement. Researchers developed the Partin Tables by analyzing thousands of pathology specimens taken at the time of surgery and comparing those results with the initial PSA levels, Gleason scores and stages.

The Partin Tables don't take into account every risk factor and cannot predict cure, but they do provide an estimate of the extent of the cancer that can help doctors and patients determine which treatment options are appropriate based on the specifics of each individual case. Patients with the highest probability that the cancer has not yet spread beyond the prostate are considered the best candidates for surgery as well as other curative treatment options such as radiation therapy. Calculations based on the Partin Tables for any individual patient are not 100% accurate, but they do provide us with a valuable assessment of the probability as to how far the cancer may have spread based on a large number of patients.

The Partin Tables are available through the Prostate Cancer Research Institute's web site located at www.pcri.org, and are part of a computer software application called Prostate Cancer Tools II. This web site provides a number of related tools—tables, nomograms and algorithms—that can help a patient analyze the likely outcomes of his specific case with regard to not only the surgical option but also with regard to external beam radiation therapy, brachytherapy, and various combination therapies that are discussed later in this book.

CHAPTER FOUR

TREATMENT OPTIONS

What are the Most Common Treatments for Prostate Cancer?

The various treatment alternatives for prostate cancer are at present classified as "curative" or "palliative." Those patients who have early stage prostate cancer are candidates for curative treatments. In the past, the treatment options for such patients had been limited to surgery (radical prostatectomy) and radiation therapy, like that used with many other forms of cancer. Both treatment modalities have seen significant advances in recent years. In addition, a number of other techniques have been developed for the treatment of early stage prostate cancer. These include cryosurgery and therapies using protons and neutrons. While some therapies remain investigational, these more recent developments have given men a wider range of alternatives than ever before.

Those patients with late stage disease, or disease that has spread beyond the prostate gland, are generally considered incurable using presently available techniques. Some of you reading this book may fall into this category. But if you have late stage prostate cancer, there is no reason to give up hope simply because the medical community presently considers your condition incurable. Prostate cancer is often a very unpredictable disease, and the fact is that many men even with metastatic disease have lived for a decade or more with little or no progression of the cancer. Many eventually die of natural causes. And there are even the rare instances of spontaneous remission.

More importantly for patients with late stage prostate cancer, there are several treatment options including hormonal therapies that can be successfully used to slow or halt progression of the disease and to alleviate symptoms. Experimentation into the efficacy of a wide array of drugs and anti-cancer agents is also underway, any one of which may turn out to be the key to an improved form of treatment. And as research continues, one day in the not too distant future we may very well find a cure for any and all stages of prostate cancer.

A comprehensive list of treatment options and guidelines for cancer care professionals has been published by the National Comprehensive Cancer Network (NCCN), which includes specialists from 19 leading medical centers in the U.S. The guidelines are available from the American Cancer Society's National Cancer Information Center (1-800-ACS-2345), from the ACS web site (www.cancer.org) and the NCCN telephone information center (1-888-909-NCCN).

What Should a Patient Consider When Choosing a Treatment?

To get a handle on the basics of your case, you will need to find out from your doctor the following: 1) how much cancer you have, 2) where the cancer is located, and 3) how aggressive the cancer is. After your cancer has been graded and staged, you still have a lot to consider before deciding on treatment. As you begin to weigh your options with your doctor, you will want to take into account the following:

- ✔ Your age and life expectancy.
- ✔ Your overall health and any other serious medical conditions you may have.
- ✔ The stage, grade and risk factors associated with your cancer.
- ✔ The likelihood of cure with each type of treatment.
- ✔ Your concerns about the possible side effects associated with treatment.

Deciding on the best treatment and choosing the right doctor can be difficult. There are a number of legitimate treatment options, and each has its pros and cons. A persuasive argument can often be made for more than one option for which you may be eligible. To choose between treatments, you should carefully consider the likelihood of cure and the potential complications of each form of therapy. These are objective factors, but there are also equally important subjective factors relating to your personality, your priorities, emotional needs, and lifestyle.

Again, it is important to emphasize that each patient is different. Some men are extremely uncomfortable with the idea of having to live with side effects after treatment. Others are more concerned with survival issues than they are with quality of life considerations. You will want to find a balance that meets your personal needs and expectations. Ideally, your doctor will tailor a treatment plan that will minimize the impact of the disease while sparing you as much as possible from undesirable side effects of therapy.

In order to have confidence in your doctor's experience and expertise, you will need to find out how many patients he has treated and what his results have been with patients who are your age and have your PSA level and Gleason score. Your doctor should also be willing to provide you with a list of patients you can contact whose cases are similar to yours and who have undergone the type of treatment you are considering. He might even invite you to his clinic where you can question patients of various ages about their cases and freedom from relapse. You might ask them if they would do it again if they had the choice today. Even with today's increased emphasis on privacy issues with regard to healthcare, many patients are willing to share their experiences with fellow patients. A doctor is more likely to refer you to men that he has treated successfully rather than to failures. But if you attend a support group meeting, you can ask those patients about their experiences with a particular treatment and/or a particular doctor. Support group contact information and additional questions for your doctor are provided in the appendices of this book.

As you chart your course, keep accurate records of your lab tests and the results of all medical and therapeutic procedures. Making lists of your priorities and concerns about treatment can also be very useful. In the end, after learning all you can about your individual case and the pros and cons of each treatment, you should be able to make an educated decision about which treatment will be right for you. Keep in mind that each type of treatment is irreversible – once you have been treated, you can't undo it, so it's worth making every effort to think it through clearly from the beginning. In this situation, you are the one who ultimately has to be comfortable with the choice you make.

How are Treatments Compared?

As mentioned earlier, there are no modern randomized trials that compare the mainstream treatments like surgery, brachytherapy (radioactive implants) and external radiation. Instead, we rely on uncontrolled retrospective comparisons using PSA and Gleason categories to stratify patient groups according to low, intermediate and high risk; and then we compare the effectiveness of the various modalities. This represents a fairly reasonable form of analysis, given the overall prognostic consistency between institutions since the advent of the PSA test.

It should be emphasized that we are evaluating reported data and not mere opinions. It's true that the data requires interpretation, and statistics can be distorted to support a particular argument or specialty. But as more data is reported involving larger numbers of patients and longer follow-up (10 and 12 year studies), the areas where distortion and disagreement come into play are increasingly limited. As time goes on, the data becomes more and more persuasive. For example, there is a growing consensus among doctors that external radiation, brachytherapy and radical prostatectomy have about the same cure rates for the earliest stage prostate cancers, as demonstrated with those patients classified as low risk. While the cure rates may be comparable with this group of patients, the likelihood of side effects vary with each type of treatment, and therefore, quality of life also becomes an important consideration.

In comparing treatments, there is at least a grain of truth to the idea that we are dealing with an apples/oranges dilemma. Because each treatment modality has its own specific rationale and methodology, the reported results need to be scrutinized carefully, as each therapeutic specialty has its own criteria for measuring success and failure (see below "What is the definition of cure?"). Historically, there has been a bias in the medical literature and news media favoring surgery, but as we will see in the pages ahead, the most recent trends supported by the data have shifted the balance in favor of radiation, especially for intermediate and high risk patients.

You should also be aware that although statistics provide a general picture of what to expect from treatment, they may not be representative of present success rates. Over the past decade, improvements in all fields have increased the effectiveness of treatment. In some cases, the reported results may be out of date and not reflect the most recent innovations. For example, external radiation therapy has advanced in terms of accuracy and effectiveness as the technology has progressed from traditional external beam radiation therapy (EBRT) to 3-dimensional conformal radiation therapy (3-D CRT), both of which have been surpassed in just the past few years by 4-Dimensional Image-Guided Intensity Modulated Radiation Therapy (4D IG-IMRT). Yet all three forms of radiation are still being utilized, and you will want to be sure exactly which type is offered by your doctor.

Finally, statistics are based on probabilities involving large numbers of patients. But as an individual, you are unique. And your case is just as unique. This is especially true when dealing with a disease as unpredictable as prostate cancer. There is always a possibility that what is true of most men may not be true for you.

What is the Definition of Cure?

Being cured of prostate cancer basically means the patient's entire cancer has been permanently eradicated. In practice, the methods that we use to determine which patients are cured have changed over the years. Before the advent of PSA monitoring, the only way for doctors to know whether any cancer was still present after treatment was if cancer was detected with a digital rectal examination or by repeated biopsies, or if metastases were found on a bone scan. With these limited means for determining the presence of cancer, many patients were mistakenly considered to be cured, when in fact they had residual cancers that were too small to be detected.

Patients whose cancers shrink after treatment to the point that they are undetectable are often described as being "in remission." But being in remission is not the same as being cured, because there is still some chance that these patients will have a recurrence of their cancer at some point in the future. Because prostate cancer progresses slowly, many patients in remission will die of other causes before their prostate cancer has time to re-grow. Before PSA testing, we couldn't be sure that a patient was really cured until about 10 to 15 years after treatment.

Since the introduction of PSA monitoring, we have been able to detect residual cancers much sooner after treatment. PSA results also showed us that cure rates were actually lower than previously believed for surgery and radiation, because of the number of residual cancers that had not been de-tected. This unexpected finding brought about a reappraisal of the entire field of prostate cancer therapy in the 1990s, at the same time spurring renewed progress by researchers working to improve the effectiveness of each type of treatment.

Soon after surgery, radiation therapy and other potential treatments, a patient's PSA will usually become undetectable or fall to very low levels. Most patients appear to be in remission shortly after being treated by any one of these curative therapies. The success of any treatment depends on achieving and maintaining a very low PSA endpoint. Some patients, how-ever, will eventually show a rising PSA level if there is residual cancer. Such a PSA relapse is known as *biochemical failure*. Most patients who have resid-ual cancer will show a rising PSA within five years of treatment. Most men whose PSA does not rise after five years are considered cured, but some ad-

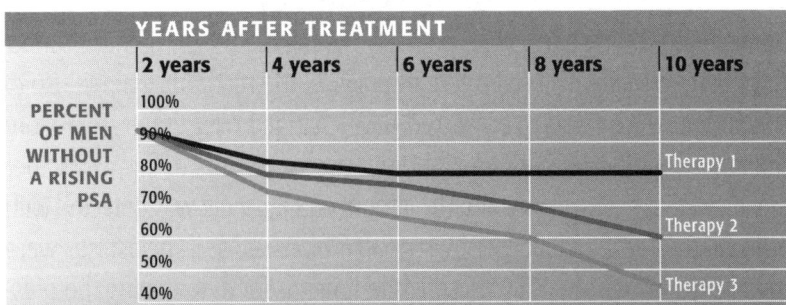

Figure 6–A graph showing the likelihood of biochemical disease survival for three hypothetical prostate cancer treatments as indicated by PSA. In this example, patients who underwent Therapy 1 showed a leveling off or plateau after about 5 years of treatment, indicating a cure rate of approximately 80%. Patients who were treated with Therapies 2 and 3 failed to plateau and continued to show additional men failing even 10 years after treatment, with the cure rate of Therapy 3 falling under 50%.

ditional men may experience a rising PSA even many years after treatment. A PSA rise following any treatment may be ominous since recurrent tumors are typically far more aggressive than the initially treated tumor.

The ultimate cure rates for each treatment modality may take many years to determine. Cure rates are often illustrated by graphs showing the percentage of men without a rising PSA over time. The cure rate is established when we see the line of the graph flatten or "plateau" after a certain number of years, indicating a percentage of men who are most likely cured by a particular type of therapy (Figure 6). The medical term for this rigorous definition of cure is *biochemical disease-free survival* (bNED).

In actual practice, doctors often define cure using different PSA values for the endpoint or *nadir* level that should be reached after successful treatment. This discrepancy needs to be taken into account when interpreting the results for each type of therapy as reported by teams of researchers at different institutions. The specific PSA nadir values and definition of cure with each treatment modality will be noted in the pages ahead as we discuss each treatment option in more detail.

How does Treatment Affect Quality of Life?

In addition to cure rates, the efficacy of treatment is also evaluated in terms of the risk of complications, also referred to as *morbidity* or *toxicity*. All treatments for prostate cancer carry some risk of side effects that can have an impact on a patient's lifestyle or quality of life (QOL). Side effects may be temporary or permanent. By following up with patients after treatment through interviews and/or questionnaires, researchers attempt to measure the effects of therapy on lifestyle.

A common complication after treatment is erectile dysfunction, often referred to as impotence. Defined in practical terms as the inability to maintain an erection sufficient for intercourse, erectile dysfunction is a potential side effect from any therapy used to treat the prostate. The problem may be caused by damage to the nerves, blood vessels or tissues that normally allow the penis to fill with blood to form an erection. Many patients who have no ejaculate (after surgery) or diminished ejaculate (after radiation) mistakenly consider themselves to be impotent.

Any large study of patients with long-term follow-up should take into account normal, age-related impotence, as there is a 2.0 % spontaneous decrease in potency with each year after the age of 40 (at age 40 only 80% have complete erectile function), and this is without any type of prostate treatment. Evaluating the effect of treatment on erectile function is made more problematical by the fact that prostate cancer typically affects an older age group for which there is a high incidence of sexual dysfunction prior to treatment. As many as 50% of prostate cancer patients already suffer from erectile dysfunction at the time they are diagnosed.

Another potential side effect of treatment is urinary incontinence, which may be caused by damage to the urethra, the bladder, and/or muscles that control urination. Temporary incontinence is common, though some men experience permanent problems. Both the risk of urinary complications and the particular symptoms vary considerably depending on the type of treatment. Fortunately, there are a number of remedies available for correcting or managing both erectile dysfunction and incontinence, thus enabling many men to maintain their quality of life after treatment.

CHAPTER FIVE

RADICAL SURGERY

What is a Radical Prostatectomy?

Unlike the simple prostatectomy performed in severe cases of BPH to remove excess tissue (an uncommon procedure today), a radical prostatectomy (RP) involves the complete removal of the prostate gland, as well as the seminal vesicles and the lymph nodes around the prostate. To the layman, the prostate is a small organ that would seem to require relatively minor surgery to remove, but due to its location, a radical prostatectomy is actually quite formidable, rivaled only by the removal of the pancreas and tongue base. The procedure may take up to four hours to perform, and because there are numerous blood vessels in the area of the prostate, the operation usually entails considerable loss of blood. Patients are encouraged to donate their blood in the weeks before the operation. Postoperative care usually involves a hospital stay from 4 to 10 days, after which the patient can go home.

There are two major forms of radical prostatectomy, based on whether a "retropubic" or "perineal" surgical technique is used. The *radical retropubic prostatectomy* is the most common form of the operation, offering the advantage of allowing for the examination of pelvic lymph nodes at the beginning of the procedure. Although diagnostic tests for identifying cancer in the lymph nodes have improved in recent years, only removal and examination of the lymph nodes can verify the presence or absence of cancer. This is important since involvement of the lymph nodes means the patient is no longer a candidate for cure using a radical prostatectomy.

Once the surgeon sees the cancer has spread to the lymph nodes, the operation is most often aborted and alternative treatment options will be considered (often radiation and/or hormonal therapy).

During the operation, the patient is first anesthetized, and a long vertical incision is made in the lower abdomen, from the navel to the pubic bone. Once the incision is made, the surgeon will routinely dissect the pelvic lymph nodes for microscopic examination. The removed lymph nodes are immediately sent to a pathologist for a "frozen section" analysis, a procedure that takes about twenty minutes. The pathologist sends the results back to the surgeon. If the lymph nodes contain microscopic evidence of cancer, the pathologist will notify the surgeon, who will then decide whether to abort or proceed with the procedure.

Most urologists believe that there is little rationale for putting the patient through the operation with no chance of cure. However, some believe that if there is only minor involvement of the lymph nodes, removal of the primary tumor in the prostate may be of some advantage for the patient in reducing symptoms of the disease and extending the patient's life. Studies done at the Mayo Clinic have demonstrated that patients undergoing RP who have diploid prostate cancer fare well with hormonal therapy and that the removal of the prostate affords a significant survival advantage. Only a very limited sampling of the lymph nodes can be removed and examined by the pathologist before the surgeon proceeds with the operation. Considerable time is spent examining lymph node samples and surgical margins ("frozen sections").

If no cancer is found by the pathologist, the operation can proceed. Access to the prostate is gained by going behind the pubic bone (hence, the name "retropubic"). The removal of the prostate is begun just above the external urethral sphincter. The prostatic urethra is divided, and the prostate is surgically removed, along with the seminal vesicles behind the bladder. The bladder neck is cut and the prostate is removed in its entirety. Then the bladder neck is pulled down and stitched to the severed end of the urethra. The larger internal sphincter must be sacrificed. This is important since it is the internal sphincter that is primarily responsible for continence, and regardless of which form of prostatectomy is performed (including minimally invasive radical prostatectomies discussed below), the large internal sphincter must be removed.

During this final phase of the operation, a catheter (a ¼ inch flexible tube) is inserted into the penis, and up into the bladder to control drainage of urine. The abdominal incision is stitched up, completing the operation. The catheter remains in place for about three weeks, and is removed on a return visit to the doctor's office.

A *radical perineal prostatectomy* approaches the prostate through the perineum, the area between the scrotum and the anus. The procedure is as potentially curative as the retropubic approach, although long-term survival data is not available. The principle advantage of the perineal technique is that the postoperative recovery is much easier on the patient. However, this procedure does not allow for the dissection and examination of lymph nodes. As a consequence, most urologists reserve this technique for those with small, localized tumors, in which the likelihood of cancerous lymph nodes is very small. Some surgeons who use the perineal approach first perform an exploratory lymphadenectomy. After a few days, if the pathologist's report indicates that the lymph nodes are free of cancer, the surgeon performs the prostatectomy.

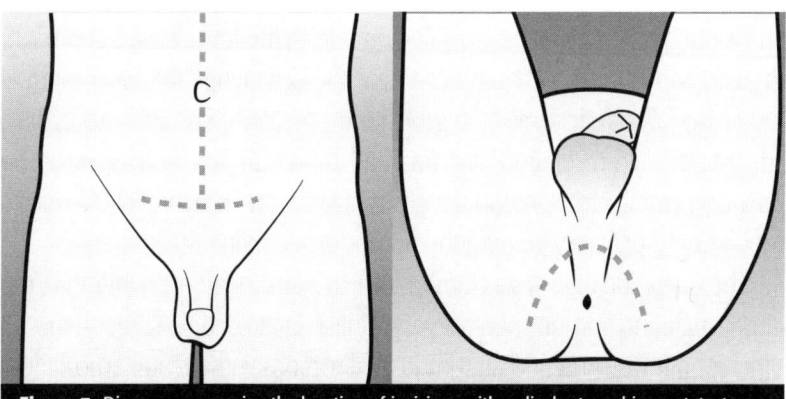

Figure 7–Diagrams comparing the location of incisions with radical retropubic prostatectomy (left) and perineal prostatectomy (right).

What are Laparoscopic Radical Prostatectomy (LRP) and the Da Vinci Robotic System?

Both of the radical procedures (RRP and RPP) described above utilize an "open" surgical technique, which involves making a long incision in order for the surgeon to remove the prostate. Minimally invasive radical prostatectomy (MIRP) is an approach that has gained popularity in recent years. One surgical technique, known as laparoscopic radical prostatectomy (LRP), employs a number of smaller incisions and special laparoscopic instruments to remove the prostate.

Laparoscopic radical prostatectomy offers certain advantages over conventional radical prostatectomy, including less blood loss and pain, shorter hospital stays, and faster recovery times, although the procedure takes longer to perform (the risks of which are discussed below). Although the laparoscopic prostatectomy is a technically challenging procedure, according to its proponents, in experienced hands, LRP may be considered comparable to the open radical procedure.

Early studies report that the rates of side effects from LRP are similar to the side effect profile obtained with open prostatectomy. A "nerve-sparing" approach is possible with LRP, possibly increasing the chance of normal erections after the operation (see below, "What are the risks of erectile dysfunction after radical surgery?").

Some surgeons do LRP remotely and indirectly by use of a robotic interface known as the da Vinci system. The procedure is gaining popularity and is often called a robotic prostatectomy. With this less invasive approach, the surgeon is seated at a console near the operating table and controls a number of robotic arms to perform the operation. The da Vinci system consists of high-resolution cameras and micro-surgical instruments. The da Vinci prostatectomy computer scales the surgical movements to micro-movements, precisely guiding the robotic arms during the surgery.

The operation involves a number of 1 to 2 cm. incisions, rather than the large single incision of open surgery. Unlike laparoscopic surgery, the da Vinci robotic instruments can turn in all directions with greater articulation. Proponents of the da Vinci system suggest that it provides the surgeon with improved visualization, dexterity, and precision compared with open or laparoscopic surgery. The robotic-assisted procedure also attempts to spare the nerves controlling bladder and sexual function.

LRP and robotic prostatectomy are not new treatments, but rather modern versions of radical prostatectomy. Because they are relatively new ways of performing the surgery, long-term studies are not yet available. While the instrumentation of LRP and the da Vinci system may allow for greater precision, they do not allow the surgeon to use the sense of touch while operating. Early studies suggest a high rate of positive surgical margins. By increasing the duration of the procedure, the laparoscopic/robotic techniques may also increase potential complications (blood clots to the lungs, infection). Most importantly, recent studies suggest a three-fold failure rate increase over open radical prostatectomy (27.8% versus 9.1%) at only 6 months (*Journal Clin Oncol,* 26: 2278-2284, May 10, 2008). Many laparoscopic/robotic procedures are aborted and converted to the more formal open approach when blood vessels are nicked or the rectum is lacerated.

It should be noted that the limitations of the open radical prostatectomy also apply to the laparoscopic and robotic approaches: the operation is necessarily performed "in the blind," in the sense that the patient's workup does not allow the surgeon to know with certainty in advance whether or not the cancer has spread beyond the prostate gland. In other words, the risk of having positive surgical margins is the same regardless of which surgical technique is used. Even the 9.1% failure rate at only 6 months with open radical prostatectomy in the study cited above calls into question the efficacy of surgical removal of the prostate by any means. One study by the University of California-Irvine reported the rate of positive surgical margins with laparoscopic radical prostatectomy as 35.5% (Ahlering TE, et al, *J Urol.* 2003 Nov;170(5):1738-41).

A more recent survey from the Memorial Sloan-Kettering Cancer Center compared the published results of LRP with retropublic radical prostatectomy (RRP) and reported as follows: "The 5-year biochemical recurrence rates range from 70-92% for the RRP vs. 82-91% for the LRP. The global positive surgical margin rates are 12-20% for the RRP and 17-30% for the LRP" (Romero-Otero J, et al, "Laparoscopic radical prostatectomy: Contemporary comparison with open surgery," *Urol. Oncol.* 2007 Nov-Dec;25(6):499-504). In my opinion, these results are far from acceptable given the attendant side effects.

If you are thinking about treatment with open radical surgery (under a surgeon's hands) or LRP or robotic-assisted radical surgery, be sure to find a surgeon with a proven track record rather than a surgeon who is just starting out with any particular technique. Experience is absolutely crucial, as there is an unusually arduous learning curve for mastering the newer surgical techniques. One study estimates as many as 100 procedures or more are required before a surgeon may be considered proficient (Ahlering TE, et al, *J Urol.* 2003 Nov;170(5):1738-41).

Which Patients are Candidates for Surgery?

Radical prostatectomy is intended as a curative treatment, and thus usually only patients with early stage prostate cancer (organ-confined disease, stages T1 and T2) are candidates for the operation. A prostatectomy is a major operation, and because of the stress and physical impact of the procedure, most surgeons discourage men older than 70 from having the operation. Because of the high risk of complications with surgery, younger men with other serious medical conditions such as heart disease are also discouraged from undergoing radical surgery.

What are the Risks of the Operation?

A prostatectomy involves some of the risks of complications that accompany any major operation. These include death associated with anesthesia, heart attack, stroke, the formation of blood clots in the legs or lungs, and infections. Fortunately, the likelihood of these complications is very small, less than 1%. Rectal damage occurs in about 1% of patients. The most common, serious complications of surgery are urinary incontinence and erectile dysfunction (see discussion below). The skill of the surgeon can significantly reduce the risk of long-term complications resulting from the procedure.

What are the Risks of Erectile Dysfunction after Radical Surgery?

Loss of sexual function is very common after surgery, since two nerve bundles associated with erection are located laterally (right / left) to the prostate gland. They closely approximate the gland at the apex (bottom). An innovative technique, pioneered by Dr. Patrick Walsh at Johns Hopkins during the early 1980s, attempts to preserve one or both of these neurovascular bundles (NVBs) during the radical prostatectomy. In theory, this nerve-sparing technique allows more patients to retain sexual function.

However, because the technique requires shaving close to the side margins of the prostate, it is often reserved for patients whose cancer is most likely to be contained well within the capsule of the prostate.

The success of the nerve-sparing procedure depends on the age and pathologic stage of the patient undergoing the operation. In the most favorable studies by the leading "artist" surgeons, men between the age of 50 and 60 have a 75% chance of retaining erectile function. Men over the age of 70 have only a 25% chance of retaining erectile function. The nerve-sparing procedure requires a high degree of surgical skill, and the results obtained by most surgeons are not as impressive as those reported by Dr. Walsh at Johns Hopkins.

The National Cancer Institute has investigated the differences in results obtained by the premier surgical centers versus those obtained by less skilled practitioners utilizing the nerve-sparing technique. Researchers found that nearly all surgical patients were impotent, while 35% of patients were incontinent after treatment. One study reported that "published estimates from physicians of impotence following various types of radical prostatectomy [including nerve-sparing RP] may be low, since not all patients may report treatment-related complications accurately and completely to their doctors. In contrast, direct surveys of patients indicate much higher rates of postoperative sexual and urinary dysfunction" (Talcott JA, et al, National Cancer Institute 1998, Jul 15; 90 (14): 1107).

Obviously, most men have quality of life concerns, and a patient considering radical prostatectomy would be wise to ask his surgeon if he uses the nerve-sparing technique and what percentage of his patients retain erectile function. Recently developed drugs such as Viagra®, Cialis®, Levitra® and Prostatgladin E1 can be used to treat erectile dysfunction resulting from the operation, and if necessary, a penile prosthesis or other remedies may be employed. Sometimes surgery can only spare the nerves on one side of the prostate, and in the past many of these men did not retain potency. In recent years thanks to drugs like Viagra®, one side may be sufficient to allow the patient to regain some degree of potency over time.

The nerve-sparing approach has also been incorporated with varying degrees of success in the open perineal prostatectomy, as well as in the laparoscopic and robotic surgical techniques. As mentioned, these newer techniques are not yet supported by long term studies.

Some other side effects of radical prostatectomy are often not candidly discussed with patients. For example, 6 to 8 months after the operation, penile shrinkage may occur because of scar tissue or the shortening of the urethra as an outcome of the procedure. For those patients who manage to retain their potency after surgery, there is no ejaculate during orgasm because the prostate gland and seminal vesicles have been removed. Orgasms experienced without ejaculate are known as dry orgasms.

When considering the pros and cons of the various treatment options, some patients are only comfortable with the idea of attempting to remove the cancer by radical surgery. This "surgical mind-set" is understandable if only because patients usually have heard more about surgery for cancer than the other treatment options, and the notion of "cutting out the cancer" appeals to some men as the simplest solution, even though the surgical data now suggests otherwise.

For many men, it is comforting for them to know that their cancerous prostate glands will be in a jar after the surgical procedure. They may be willing to accept the potential short term and long term side effects. The problem is that while the prostate may be in a jar, this does not necessarily mean that the cancer has been removed in its entirety. When this is the case, the PSA may rise at some point after surgery even though the patient no longer has a prostate gland.

Men who are inclined this way are strongly advised to ask their physicians if their own risk factors as determined by their test results actually make them good candidates for the procedure (see below, "What misleading arguments are used to promote surgery?").

What are the Risks of Incontinence after Surgery?

The trauma to the urine passage and bladder during radical surgery causes temporary urinary incontinence (involuntary urine leakage or dripping) in all patients. Most men regain varying degrees of urinary control within several weeks to several months after the operation. Others experience permanent incontinence. Loss of bladder control ranges from mild incontinence to severe incontinence, due to permanent damage done to the urethral sphincter. In these cases, exercises, medications or the surgical placement of an artificial sphincter may be used to restore urinary control to the patient.

There are generally three types of incontinence: stress incontinence, overflow incontinence, and urgency incontinence. Men with stress incontinence, the most common type after surgery, leak urine when they cough, laugh, get up or turn quickly, or lift heavy objects. Men with overflow incontinence take a long time to urinate and have a weak or dribbling stream. Men with urgency incontinence experience a sudden need to pass urine.

There is a wide variation in the medical literature as far as the likelihood that patients will experience incontinence after surgery. The numbers may vary anywhere from 5% to 65%. This discrepancy is primarily due to the fact that doctors use different definitions to describe incontinence. If a patient has only slight leakage (for example, only one diaper daily), some doctors report that the patient is not incontinent, while other doctors consider a patient with any urine leakage to be incontinent. A realistic estimate of the likelihood of incontinence would probably be about 25% of patients with the best surgical care. On December 1, 2006, the *New York Times* reported that "up to 29 percent of men who have their prostates removed report wearing pads to keep dry, according to one large study."

Why is Hormonal Therapy sometimes used Before Surgery?

Hormonal therapy, also known as Androgen Ablation Therapy (ADT), can shrink a man's prostate up to 50%. Some surgeons recommend the use of hormonal therapy for several months prior to surgery. The rationale is that reducing the size of the prostate will make it easier to remove. While there is no definitive proof that hormonal downsizing will increase the likelihood of cure with surgery, it remains a valid option for some patients. Many surgeons discourage hormones since they believe that there is more capsular scarring, making it especially difficult to excise the gland or spare the nerve bundles. Others use hormones as a temporary regimen, allowing the patient more time to explore his treatment options without concern about cancer progression.

What are the Treatment Options If Surgery Fails?

In men who show a measurable PSA after surgery (often defined as a PSA of 0.2 or higher), the likelihood is that some cancer was left at the margins of the prostate or that some cancer may have spread to other areas of the body, even though it may not be detected by lymph node dissection or by bone scans. In these cases, further surgery is not advisable.

A second attempt at a cure with another type of treatment is called "salvage therapy," because it attempts to salvage a cure after an initial treatment failure. The common forms of salvage therapy for patients who are at risk for failure after surgery are radiation therapy and hormonal therapy. Many patients are clinically understaged—that is, they have more cancer than they are told—and are found to have *positive surgical margins* (cancer beyond the gland and outside the surgical field), or to have extracapsular extension or seminal vesicle involvement either at the time of surgery or pathologically. Some of these patients may opt for watchful waiting to see if their PSA starts rising before they decide to embark on another course of therapy.

Instead of waiting for the PSA to signal a recurrence of cancer, some urologists encourage patients in this category to begin a course of radiation therapy in the hope of avoiding problems later. This is referred to as *adjuvant radiation therapy*. Radiation is delivered to the prostatic region in the hope that it will destroy any cancer that may remain there. External radiation following surgery has been shown to reduce the risk of biochemical relapse (rising PSA) by approximately 30% (as evidenced by the fact that about 30% of men show an undetectable PSA after salvage radiation). There are many patients whose cancers are not controlled by the lower radiation doses that are typically used. This is the case since the target area becomes the void of the prostate, which is occupied by the critical bladder and rectum after surgery. In addition, radiation works best in an oxygenated field, whereas the target area after surgery is denuded and far less vascular, hence, less oxygenated. To improve matters, we use higher radiation doses with highly sophisticated radiation methods (4D IG-IMRT with DART—see Chapter Six, "Radiation Therapy"). We also combine the radiation with hormonal therapy, since the combination is superior to using only one modality. This is referred to as "synergism." To minimize the risk of complications, doctors usually allow surgical patients to recover for 3 to 6 months before starting radiation therapy.

External radiation is the most common salvage treatment for presumed local failure after surgery, while hormonal therapy is most often prescribed in cases of distant failure and evidence of metastatic disease. Some doctors favor using hormonal therapy after surgery as soon as there is any evidence of recurrence. The rationale is that hormones may slow the progress of the disease for some time. The idea of a hormonal cure is doubtful, but hormones do interrupt the spread of the disease temporarily. For some men, this knowledge may be enough to prompt them to try some form of hormonal intervention early on. Other patients may prefer to wait. Recent data, however, suggests that early hormonal intervention is superior to delayed treatment.

Depending on the particular hormone or combination of hormones that are prescribed, many men experience some side effects such as erectile dysfunction, loss of sexual desire (libido), breast enlargement, hot flashes, nausea, diarrhea, liver enzyme elevation, muscle weakness, joint aches or pains, and bone fragility (loss of bone integrity). Depending on the type of hormone prescribed, there are also a number of medications and treatment options which should be used to minimize or ameliorate these side effects. At our institution, we prefer using hormones in intermittent fashion for 6 to 12 months rather than continuous hormones. With intermittent hormonal therapy, the patient's testosterone level recovers and his quality of life (QOL) improves dramatically. The hormonal therapy is resumed once the PSA increases back to an arbitrary number (e.g., for example 5 to 10, or 10 to 15).

Patients who opt for watchful waiting after local failure with surgery must be monitored very carefully. Waiting means being prepared to treat specific symptoms of the disease with radiation and/or hormonal therapies if and when it becomes necessary to do so. As will be discussed in more detail later, hormones sooner or later will cease to be effective, though this can take many years for some men. When this occurs, the cancer is referred to as hormone refractory or hormone resistant. When hormonal therapy fails to stop the prostate cancer from spreading, the cancer may behave aggressively, with progression being imminent. In this situation, chemotherapy (cytotoxic systemic agents) may be considered (see Chapter Eight: Treating Metastatic Disease).

Why is Surgery No Longer the Treatment of Choice for Most Patients?

Historically, radical prostatectomy was for many years the primary treatment for early stage prostate cancer and most urologists regarded it as the "gold standard" treatment (and most still hang on to that belief despite data to the contrary). Since urologists are the specialists who see most prostate cancer patients after diagnosis, it is not surprising that they recommend their specialty and that in the past most patients chose the surgical option. That situation has changed in recent years with advances in alternative, non-surgical treatments such as radiation therapy. With more men being diagnosed earlier thanks to PSA screening and patients doing more research prior to embarking on a treatment course, the number of radical prostatectomies has fallen dramatically since the early 1990s. That trend is likely to continue as more patients opt for non-surgical treatments with comparable or superior cure rates and a lower risk of complications. A similar trend can be seen with breast cancer patients. It is now mandatory for breast cancer patients to consult a radiation oncologist in addition to a breast surgeon, with more women choosing lumpectomy plus radiation rather than undergoing radical mastectomy.

What Cure Rates have been Reported by the Premier Surgeons?

When comparing radical surgery with other treatment options in the PSA era, findings have been consistent when grouping patients in low, intermediate and high risk categories. With a follow-up of ten years or longer, prostatectomy appears to be effective in 80% to 90% of patients, as reported by teams from the leading specialty centers, but this success rate applies only to patients with low risk, favorable tumors (PSA < 10, Gleason score ≤ 6, clinical stage T2a or less).

With intermediate and high risk patients (PSA greater than 10, Gleason 7 to 10, clinical state equal to or greater than T2b), the data shows that these patients have a high risk for biochemical failure after radical

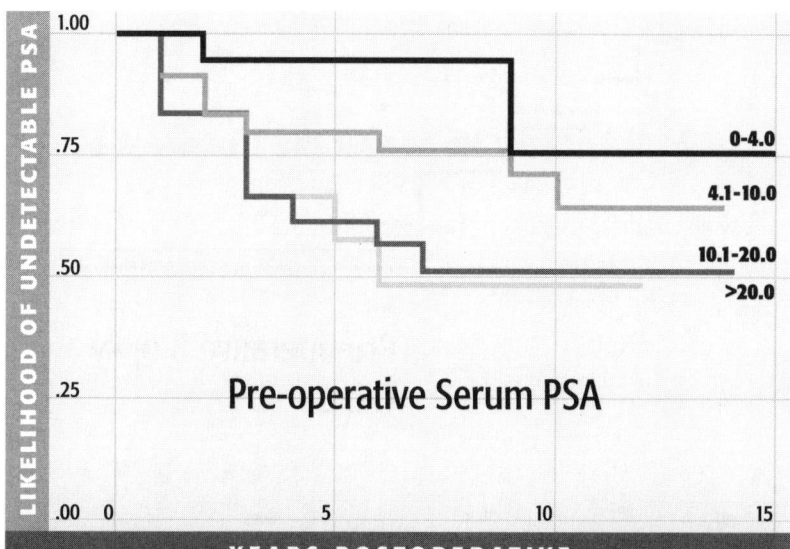

Figure 8–Likelihood of biochemical failure (rising PSA) by pre-operative serum PSA (Khan MA, Partin AW, The Oncologist, Vol. 8, No. 3, 259–269, June 2003). Data derived from the series by Dr. Patrick Walsh, Johns Hopkins Hospital, 1982-2001 (Figures 8-9). COURTESY OF *THE ONCOLOGIST*

prostatectomy. Indeed, it is with the higher risk groups that the results obtained with surgery have deteriorated to the point of being woefully unacceptable. The lack of any plateau in the disease-free survival curves of surgery patients with a pre-treatment PSA above 10 and/or a Gleason score of 7 or higher is especially striking coming from a leading institution like Johns Hopkins (see Figures 8-9). Note that these researchers defined biochemical disease-free survival after surgery as having an undetectable PSA.

What Misleading Arguments are used to Promote Surgery?

While legitimate arguments can be made for and against each type of treatment, a number of misleading arguments are often made in favor of the use of surgery over radiation. The common sense notion of "cutting the cancer out" is used to imply that a radical prostatectomy is the most effective therapy. But the fact is that 50% or more of patients with intermediate or high risk cancers will fail after surgery.

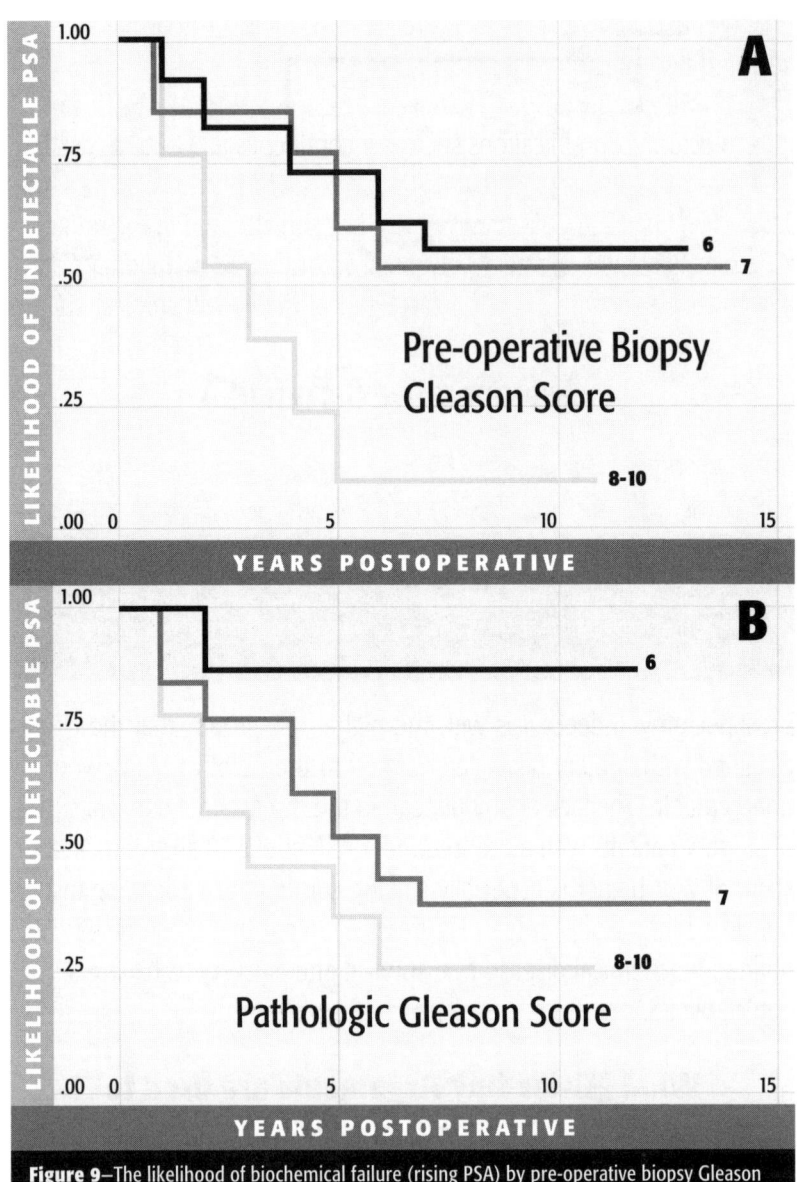

Figure 9–The likelihood of biochemical failure (rising PSA) by pre-operative biopsy Gleason score (A) and by pathologic Gleason score (B). COURTESY OF *THE ONCOLOGIST*

Another argument often used to promote surgery over radiation is the assertion that if a patient undergoes radiation and it fails, then surgery as a salvage treatment will not be an option. In fact, this is not the case. Many experienced surgeons will perform a prostatectomy at this point, albeit the operation is more difficult, as tissue that has been ir-radiated becomes more fragile. Depending on the institution reporting, between 10% and 50% of these patients can be cured by a salvage prostatectomy. Complications such as incontinence and erectile dysfunc-tion increase somewhat, and the surgeons appear to be far more willing to disclose these complications which they can attribute to the radiation. Complication rates are relatively high according to a National Cancer Institute investigation of patients treated primarily with radical surgery (without ever receiving radiation), although the surgeons appear to be less forthcoming in this regard.

Treatment options for patients who have failed radiation are actually quite numerous. In addition to a salvage prostatectomy, they may in-clude salvage brachytherapy, Intensity Modulated Radiation Therapy and brachytherapy (combined), cryosurgery and HIFU (all of which are dis-cussed in greater detail below). It is the flip side of the coin that is actu-ally more troublesome—the patient who has had surgery and fails. At this point, it is often unclear whether the PSA is rising due to local recurrence, or distant relapse (which may be microscopic and not detected by bone scans, CT scans, MRI, etc.) or both. In this situation, only salvage radiation is an option for potential cure, and recent studies demonstrate that only 10% to 30% of patients can be successfully salvaged (rescued), which is not very encouraging.

CHAPTER SIX

RADIATION THERAPY

What is Radiation and How Does It Work?

X-ray radiation is a form of energy similar to visible light. When directed at the body, x-rays penetrate tissue and are gradually absorbed. Some of the radiation is absorbed by cells and damages the DNA that normally allows cells to function and reproduce. Cancer cells are somewhat more sensitive to radiation than are healthy cells, and therefore, the radiation used to destroy cancer cells is less likely to damage normal tissues, which are tenacious. However, this difference in sensitivity is generally small and the dose of radiation required to destroy prostate cancer cells is high enough that there is some risk of damage to healthy tissue in the nearby rectum or bladder.

The strategy with radiation therapy over the years has been to deliver higher and higher doses more and more accurately to the targeted cancer, while sparing healthy adjacent tissue in order to avoid rectal and urinary complications. Since the 1950s, external radiation therapy has been a common technique used for the treatment of many kinds of cancers. It is a standard treatment for prostate cancer that is clinically confined to the prostate and surrounding tissues (stages T1, T2, and T3). It may also be prescribed for some patients whose prostate cancer that has spread to the pelvic lymph nodes. Patients with advanced prostate cancer may also be treated with external radiation as a palliative (non-curative) therapy to reduce the size of the tumor and alleviate symptoms.

What is External Beam Radiation Therapy?

With the conventional approach known as external beam radiation therapy (EBRT), high energy X-rays are targeted directly to the region of the prostate to kill or incapacitate any cancer cells in the area. The machine most widely used today to administer EBRT is the linear accelerator, which uses electrical principles (electrons) to generate photon radiation. The linear accelerator has largely replaced an older generation of machines that utilized radioactive cobalt and were not as accurate.

Radiation is given to the patient in small daily doses, usually five days a week over a course of 7 to 8 weeks. Delivering small, incremental doses over time decreases the chance of damaging healthy tissue. Radiation is completely painless and cannot be felt by the patient. Typically, a single treatment can be carried out in several minutes. Radiation is measured by a unit called the Gray (Gy), roughly analogous to a Watt of light. The old unit of measure for radiation dose rates was called the "rad", now called the centigray (cGy). 100 cGy=1 Gy unit. A typical daily dose of external radiation may range from about 180 to 200 centigray (1.8 to 2.0 Gy).

Preparation for radiation therapy is a rigorously complex process that involves exact determination of the region to receive treatment and the appropriate dose of radiation. Radiation treatments are precisely designed for each patient, because each man's prostate and surrounding organs are unique in size and shape. A planning session is carried out with the patient several days before treatments begin. In order to keep the patient in the same position for each daily treatment, he will be fitted to a custom-made mold called an "alpha cradle." Once the patient's body is properly aligned, fluoroscopic, computerized tomography ("Cone Beam Tomo Therapy"), and ultrasound imaging techniques are used to visualize the prostate and nearby organs. Even respiratory acquisition video ("Respiratory Grating") is utilized to account for small movement associated with breathing ("pelvic breathing"). The position of these critical structures will determine where the radiation beams should be directed and also the shape of the beams. The tools described above allow thorough evaluation of the 4th dimension (motion) prior to and during treatment. Adjustments are constantly made as indicated. These techniques are known as Adaptive Radiation Therapy (ART) or Dynamic Adaptive Radiation Therapy (DART). During treatment, beams from several directions converge to form a high-dose target zone, which includes the prostate and a margin of tissue surrounding the gland.

The radiation can be focused on the target area while minimizing the risk of over-radiating the rectum and bladder.

What are the Risks of Side Effects with External Radiation?

As with radical prostatectomy, there are possible side effects with external beam radiation therapy. Common side effects are fatigue, urinary urgency, frequency and burning on urination, and rectal irritation. The majority of these symptoms will disappear after treatment is concluded, but in some cases damage to the bladder or, less frequently, to the rectum results in chronic complications. These include urethral and bladder inflammation and the need to urinate more frequently (urethritis, cystitis), and intermittent periods of rectal bleeding or rectal urgency that may continue for years afterwards. Severe bladder or rectal injury is very rare using today's sophisticated technologies. Although most men retain erectile function after the conclusion of radiation therapy, as many as half of the men who undergo conventional EBRT will eventually develop erectile dysfunction.

The skill of the radiotherapist administering treatments can significantly reduce the risk of complications, as can the use of more advanced technology. Conventional EBRT has largely been replaced in this country by more sophisticated techniques for delivering radiation. As discussed below, 3-D Conformal Radiation, Intensity Modulated Radiation Therapy, and brachytherapy have shown superior results both for curing the cancer and reducing the likelihood of complications. The most advanced form of IMRT currently available is known as 4 Dimensional Image-Guided Intensity Modulated Radiation Therapy (4D IG-IMRT), with Dynamic Adaptive Radiotherapy (DART).

What is 3D-Conformal Radiation Therapy?

In the past, some researchers suggested that radiation therapy might only halt progression of the disease for a number of years, after which the cancer would recur. But many radiotherapists argued that this was only the case if the radiation beam was imprecisely directed during treatment and thus failed to deliver a sufficient cancer-killing dose. Until the mid-1980s, the maximum dose that could be safely administered to the prostate was thought to be 7000 centigray. Higher doses at that time were associated with an unacceptably high risk of complications. With the improved technologies in use today, doses of 7000 to 8000 centigray are common with the technique known as 3D-Conformal Radiation (3D-CRT), which has greatly reduced the risk of complications.

Since the mid-1980s, three-dimensional computerized imaging techniques have vastly improved the accuracy of external radiation and allowed for the safe delivery of increased doses. Guided by these technological innovations, the radiotherapist molds blocks of lead alloy to conform precisely to the outline of the tumor. In order to shield healthy tissues and organs that are to be avoided, the blocks are clamped to the end of the linear accelerator, and by this means, the radiation treatment is precisely tailored for each individual patient.

Long term results of ten years and longer with 3D-Conformal Radiation Therapy have been very favorable. Because of the increased accuracy, side effects of conformal radiation are less common than with the traditional application of external beam radiation therapy. In addition, the increased dose delivered by 3D-CRT has increased cure rates to a point comparable to those achieved with surgery. Yet even this relatively advanced technique for delivering external radiation has been surpassed by cutting edge modalities such as Intensity Modulated Radiation Therapy and brachytherapy.

Does Dose Matter?

The results of a Memorial Sloan-Kettering study that compared 5-year biochemical disease-free survival among patient risk groups receiving low dose (6480 to 7020 cGy) versus high dose (7560 to 8640 cGy). Note that higher doses showed a significant advantage for all risk groups (Zelefsky, et al).

RISK GROUP	LOW DOSE	HIGH DOSE
Low	77%	90%
Intermediate	50%	70%
High	21%	47%

What is Intensity Modulated Radiation Therapy?

Intensity Modulated Radiation Therapy (IMRT) is currently the successor to 3D-CRT, taking 3D-CRT to an even higher level of precision and control (See Color Inset Images 3-A, 3-B). With IMRT, the single beam of radiation is replaced by thousands of "beamlets" or "micro-beams," each with its own intensity, energy level and destination, as directed by the radiation oncologist. A unique treatment blueprint is mapped out in advance for each patient. With computer planning and three-dimensional imaging techniques, the physician is able to more accurately deliver radiation to satisfy pre-defined dose specifications to not only the prostate but to the tumor while avoiding nearby healthy tissue. Thus, the risk of damaging the bowel, bladder, rectum and other organs is significantly reduced. At the same time, the cancer-killing dose of radiation is maximized on the designated target.

As noted above, the most sophisticated form of IMRT is known as 4-Dimensional Image-Guided Intensity Modulated Radiation Therapy (4D IG-IMRT) with Dynamic Adaptive Radiotherapy (DART). The Dattoli Cancer Center & Brachytherapy Research Institute was the first private facility in the world to offer patients both IMRT and 4D IG-IMRT with DART. This multifaceted modality utilizes a number of advanced targeting and imaging techniques even beyond what was available just a few years ago with the first generation of IMRT. The 4th dimension refers to motion and the ability to track motion (patient and organ movement) thanks in part to enhanced imaging and computer programming capabilities.

The references to IMRT in the sections immediately ahead generally apply to the entire range of technologies currently being used, including 4D IG-IMRT, which utilizes a number of technical refinements that will be discussed in greater detail below (see "4D IG-IMRT Analysis Tools" and "What is Dynamic Adaptive Radiotherapy?").

How is IMRT Planned and Performed?

With IMRT, each treatment volume is considered on a voxel by voxel basis (with a voxel being a 3-dimensional millimeter of space, compared to a pixel which is 2-dimensional) and each voxel may receive a different dose. This is like treating an area the size of a tip of a pen. Once the "target" has been designated, a planning phase referred to as "inverse treatment planning" generates beam profiles with varying intensities across the treatment field. The intensity profile of each beamlet is adjusted to satisfy the pre-defined dose specifications to the tumor as well as to the normal tissues. A computer, using mathematical optimization algorithms, then runs the optimization program, which selects the best combination of directions and beam intensities to obtain the ideal optimized plan. The program consists of literally thousands of discreet angles and doses.

To accomplish the planning phase, extremely sophisticated computerized software is utilized and plans are generated in a time frame measured in hours. This task might take a world class physicist years to accomplish. Since we are generating high-energy beamlets at specific cubic millimeter targets, immobilization of the patient is imperative. For this reason, a number of checks and balances are put into place. For example, for each patient, a customized "alpha-cradle" (similar to a body cast or mold) is designed for immobilization of the lower body in the supine position.

Once the patient's treatment profile has been digitally reconstructed, and a specific program or "blueprint" for that patient is developed, verification of the IMRT treatment is performed by utilizing amorphous silicone diode imaging, which is referred to as "Portal Vision." This silicon diode has unprecedented resolution and image acquisition, so that the doctor can watch the treatment in "real time," or review this program at the workstation at a later time. The actual delivery of the radiation is a dynamic process and is accomplished through the use of multi-leaf collimators. These devices essentially allow us to "sculpt" the beams in order to deliver the precise dose required (see Color Inset Images 3-B, 3-C, 3-E, 3-F, 3-G, 3-H, 3-I).

4D IG-IMRT Analysis Tools for Image Guidance to Achieve DART

STRICT IMMOBILIZATION TECHNIQUES using alpha cradles, subgating cameras and the table, which is now called the "exact couch." If there is more than a millimeter of motion, that will be sensed and a default will come into play.

ELECTRONIC ONLINE PORTAL IMAGING ("Portal Vision") using amorphous silicon diode technology which allows for real-time on-line verification of patient's exact treatment plan. This is an eloquent way of looking at the patient in real time.

PORTAL DOSIMETRY allows us to identify if the patient has changed or if there is motion during the treatment period. We go out of our way to create a "virtual you," a true image of you that is an accurate blueprint. If Portal Imaging shows a change, then Portal Dosimetry will automatically re-optimize your treatment plan.

ELECTRONIC ON-BOARD IMAGING for real-time evaluation.

CONE BEAM CT ("Tomo Therapy") involves real-time helical CT anatomical reconstruction of patient's anatomy to determine the actual daily delivered dose (also for "Adaptive Radiotherapy"). This is an actual CT Cone Beam activated while the patient is being treated. Digital images are reconstructed by cone beam every 102 milliseconds (much like a camera with a rapid shutter speed). We have a wireless real time system that enables physicians to watch what is happening with the patient in real time. We watch the treatment, and if we don't like what is happening, we hit a button. So there is still the human touch to all of this advanced technology.

It should be noted that Cone Beam CT ("Tomo Therapy") is not the same as "tomotherapy." The latter is actually a form of radiation treatment delivered using CT guidance, both of which are continuous in nature and very slow (rotational arc). The patient is often treated for 40 minutes so that the "BEAM-ON TIME" is enormous. This leads to "incident planned radiation," which then has a high integral dose because of the arc and the duration of treatment, with scattered photons and neutrons from the planned incident radiation, and the radiation from a continuously revolving CT Scan, which can also impart a sizeable dose to the entire body. As such, with this form of radiation treatment, there is a high risk of developing secondary cancers. Indeed, tomotherapy delivers such enormous doses of Total Body Radiation that it is not recommended in pediatric cancers (patients in their twenties or less). Why would a 50 year old or even a 60 year old patient want to undergo tomotherapy for prostate cancer only to get leukemia after 5 to 10 years?

In contrast, at our institution, we use "light speed" CT scans for diagnostics, which is accomplished in seconds. Our Cone Beam CT is also a "light speed" scanner so that the radiation dose is quantifiable although small and safe. The problem is that Cone Beam CT is often referred to as "Cone Beam CT Tomo Therapy," but it is really Cone Beam (CB) *Tomography*. It is not a form of treatment, but just one of our many image guidance tools used in conjunction with 4D IG-IMRT and DART (see "What is Dynamic Adaptive Radiotherapy?").

REAL-TIME 4D REVIEW by physicians using wireless network system which conveys images to remote tablet.

SONARRAY® 3D VIRTUAL ULTRASOUND ACQUISITION with remote capabilities, Optical Camera Based Tracking Subsystem for immediate system default. This technique allows for intra-fractional motion gating for Dynamic Adaptive Radiation Therapy (DART). This allows us to check before treatment for the amount of fluid in the bladder and air in the rectum. The Optical Camera tracking system then follows the patient, and if at any moment he moves, there is an automatic default. We have infrared lasers scanning the body, so if the patient moves, there is a default. With video acquisition respiratory cameras watching the patient, he may cough and that will be tracked and immediately, the beam will be turned off, so the patient doesn't have to worry if he moves during the 4D IG-IMRT treatment process.

RESPIRATORY GATING is another way that we can identify patient motion, with advanced video tracking technology which allows for real-time monitoring and correction of physiologic motion of prostate which may occur as a result of patient breathing (also for Dynamic Adaptive Radiation Therapy).

Daily localization of the target is essential to optimize therapeutic effects since both patient and organ movement may occur. It should be noted that all of the techniques described above (4D IG-IMRT Analysis Tools) are non-invasive. These routines are implemented with comprehensive checklists that are crucial to ensure accurate targeting on a daily basis.

At the Dattoli Cancer Center, most patients are treated Monday through Friday for approximately four to five weeks. They are seen daily by the radiation technologists and at least once a week by a nurse as well as the doctor as indicated. After completion of the IMRT, many patients return in three to six weeks for brachytherapy, if their risk factors mandate a combined approach. After seed implantation, they may also receive a short follow-up course of several additional IMRT treatments to sterilize any microscopic cancer that might remain in peri-prostatic tissues or lymph nodes (while carefully avoiding the prostate).

What is Dynamic Adaptive Radiotherapy (DART)?

For more than four decades, the evolution of radiation delivery technologies has been based upon a single objective: maximize the dose to the tumor while minimizing the dose to surrounding normal tissue (thereby minimizing side effects). Today, using 4D IG-IMRT, physicians are able to realize the full potential of what is known as "Dynamic Adaptive Radiotherapy" (DART).

DART is a coordinated systems approach made possible by the technological convergence of image-guided tools, which integrate both image and data management while utilizing sophisticated treatment planning capabilities such as "autosegmentation" and "deformable registration"—all for the purpose of optimized IMRT treatment delivery. Such a cutting edge system ties together every step, from 4D IG-IMRT simulation and treatment planning to adaptive treatment delivery based on the reality of a patient's exact treatment "condition" and position each and every day, as it changes. Doctors are aware that changes such as tumor position, size and shape do occur not only during a several week treatment regime, but also on a daily basis.

DART achieves the single most important goal ever achieved in radiation therapy, by delivering the exact dose to the exact place at exactly the precise time, every time, even when the target moves, shrinks or changes shape—an extraordinary accomplishment!

The actual implementation of DART relies on handling large volumes of continuously changing patient data, interpreting those changes and then immediately acting upon them in real-time. For example, rather than using a one-size-fits-all approach, physicians are empowered to choose a dose schema (e.g. "boost") at a chosen moment in time and make necessary changes to a treatment plan "on the fly" based on cone-beam image capture that reveals real-time changes in the target as it responds to treatment. The bottom line involves managing the motion and biological changes of the target (tumor) and dynamically adapting the 4D IG-IMRT treatment. This makes for truly "individualized" treatment delivery.

Although each individual is unique, at the Dattoli Cancer Center & Brachytherapy Research Institute, most patients being treated receive a treatment protocol of combination therapy, utilizing 4-D IG-IMRT and seed implantation (brachytherapy). Both of these state-of-the art treatment modalities rely on advanced imaging techniques and sophisticated computer software programs.

The resurgence of interest in prostate brachytherapy over the past two decades was primarily driven by the technological innovation of transrectal ultrasound (TRUS), which allows for real time imaging during treatment planning and is also used for monitoring intraoperative needle placement. TRUS imaging is supplemented by computerized tomography (CT) and endorectal magnetic resonance imaging (MRI). Each imaging modality has its advantages and disadvantages.

TRUS, MRI and CT images all reveal pre-treatment prostate contours and can be used in tandem to determine the number and placement of implant seeds (ie. Palladium-103, Iodine-125). While the appearance of the prostatic and periprostatic regions varies qualitatively between the imaging modalities, the size and shape of the prostate are fairly consistent between techniques when interpreted correctly.

The visualization of prostate margins with these complementary modalities ultimately determines the radioactivity required and where it is placed. The same holds true for 4D IG-IMRT, which is often combined with seeding as the protocol of choice for intermediate and higher risk patients. The most advanced imaging technologies now being utilized in conjunction with IMRT include Varian 4D IG-IMRT technology with SonArray Ultrasound-Guided Positioning, Online Portal Vision Imagery, Cone Beam Tomography, Respiratory Grating, and real-time 4D physician review. These technologies allow for the checks and balances necessary to deliver DART most effectively.

How does IMRT Compare to 3D-CRT and What Kind of IMRT is the Best Currently Available?

While IMRT is not yet widely used outside of major medical centers, recent studies comparing IMRT to 3D-CRT have demonstrated a very significant advantage for IMRT with respect to both success rates and reduction of side effects. One study from Memorial Sloan-Kettering showed IMRT increased the success rate in shrinking tumors from 43% to 96%, while decreasing complications from 10% to 2%. Our IMRT team and others are reporting similar findings.

As we will see in the pages ahead, 4D IG-IMRT offers even greater advantages when it is combined with brachytherapy, especially with intermediate and high risk patients. It should also be noted that 4D IG-IMRT is not considered an experimental procedure, but is rather the culmination of earlier external radiation delivery systems. Like brachytherapy, 4D-IG IMRT is both FDA and Medicare approved, and its effectiveness has already been demonstrated by many scientific studies.

Keep in mind that with the rapid advances in IMRT and related technologies, not all IMRT is created equal. Many institutions advertize that they offer "IMRT" when in fact they have only early generations of this technology. *Patients are strongly advised to make sure their doctors are equipped with the latest IMRT technology, namely 4D IG-IMRT with DART.* By taking the time to locate which medical centers in their area have state of the art technology, patients are more likely to have successful outcomes. Many patients travel to our center from around the world simply because we have the most advanced technology and we are continually upgrading to maintain the highest standards.

Which Patients are Eligible for External Radiation Therapy?

Because external radiation (EBRT, 3D-CRT, and IMRT) is non-invasive and does not require an operation or anesthesia, most men can safely tolerate this form of therapy. The likelihood of cure is greatest with low risk patients (clinical stage T1, non-palpable tumors, less than 50% core involvement found in the biopsy specimens, a Gleason score $\leq$ 6, serum PSA $\leq$

10, and a non-elevated PAP). Intermediate and high risk patients can also be effectively treated with external radiation (preferable 4D IG-IMRT), but more favorable results for these patients are now being achieved when external radiation is combined with brachytherapy.

With the combined protocol of 4D IG-IMRT and brachytherapy, even patients having locally advanced disease with regional lymph node involvement have enjoyed long disease-free intervals and even a cure. These patients were previously thought to be incurable. In addition, patients with metastatic disease beyond the regional lymph nodes have not been considered curable in the past; however, with the most recent advances in technology, we are beginning to push the envelope with our ability to treat more advanced cases. We are now able to treat the primary tumor, and with certain limitations, we can treat all known sites of metastatic deposits to prolong the disease-free interval.

In patients having metastatic disease, when the cancer in the prostate region is causing urinary or rectal problems, they are often treated with external radiation. Patients with bone metastases may also receive radiation to relieve pain.

What is RapidArc™ and Does it Offer Advantages for IMRT System Delivery?

According to the manufacturer, Varian Medical Systems, RapidArc™ is a technological innovation that promises to deliver a complete IMRT treatment with a single rotation of the treatment machine around the patient. This technology is known as "volumetric modulated arc therapy," and the advantage touted by the company is that treatment time may be 2 to 10 times faster than earlier generations of IMRT, including 4D IG-IMRT. RapidArc™ has been licensed by the FDA and is being aggressively marketed. In order to incorporate RapidArc™, a fully realized IMRT system must be in place along with a patient information management system known as Aria™. RapidArc™ is a very costly endeavor that initially sounds promising, but the reality is that with arc therapy of this kind, the integral dose will be higher with a continuous open beam (arc) of radiation directed at the patient. That high integral dose rate may have the potential of increasing secondary malignancies in the long term.

The selling point with RapidArc™ for the manufacturer is that patients can be treated more quickly with a smaller support staff. The crucial question is what the dose rate should be in order to safely eradicate cancer while sparing healthy tissue. I have serious reservations about this technology because changing the dose rate in this way could lead to deleterious outcomes with IMRT over time. To date, there are no clinical toxicity studies of RapidArc™. It may be that in the future, arc therapy will be segmented to address these issues; but for the time being, at our institution, we have decided not to incorporate this technology in our 4D IG-IMRT system arsenal because of our concerns about the high dose rate. We are not yet convinced that it will be effective and not have detrimental late effects. Further long term studies are warranted and patients are advised to exercise caution with healthcare providers who sing the praises of RapidArc™. Once again, what is "new" is not necessarily "better."

What is the Calypso 4D® System and how does it compare to 4D IG-IMRT?

The Calypso® 4D Localization System is an attempt to address the problem of organ motion in external radiation therapy. According to the manufacturer, "Calypso Medical has developed a platform to objectively locate the tumor and monitoring tumor motion accurately and continuously without adding ionizing radiation. The Calypso® 4D Localization System consists of three components: the Calypso® 4D Localization System located in the treatment room; the Calypso® 4D Tracking Station located in the control room and Beacon® transponders, which are small wireless electromagnetic circuits designed for permanent implantation in the body. The Beacon transponders interact with the Calypso System and locate tumor's position, guide the therapist to setup the treatment…" (from the Calypso Medical Web site–http://www.calypsomedical.com/news/presskit_files/presskit_organmotion.pdf).

In comparing the Calypso® 4D System with 4D IG-IMRT with DART, it is important to keep in mind that our Varian 4D IG-IMRT with DART system is an integrated system that is a fully interfaced piece of equipment that delivers precise dosing of radiation to intraprostatic sites as well as periprostatic margin and affected lymph nodes. 4D IG-IMRT accomplished all of this in addition to accounting for organ motion in real time during the actual treatment, as well as real time dose optimization to intensify dose to specific targeted areas. It adjusts for dose to identified areas spontaneously while de-modulating or lessening the dose to surrounding critical structures.

Calypso, on the other hand, is essentially a piece of equipment that can be adapted to any existing linear accelerator. The Calypso system functions much like a gold seed marker in the prostate. Little electromagnetic transponders (called beacons) are placed into the prostate (2-3 of them) and they serve as a localization technique to track where the prostate is. It is then up to the radiation therapists delivering the treatment to identify if the target is not being treated appropriately and the patient needs to be moved. This is not near the sophistication of an integrated system like 4D IG-IMRT, and can only account for prostate mobility. It cannot account for movement and identification of surrounding critical structures such as bladder and rectum, not to mention penile vessel anatomy, penile bulb, etc.

What is the Cyberknife® Robotic Radiosurgery System?

The Cyberknife® is essentially a linear accelerator mounted on a robotic arm. This modality was developed at Stanford in the 1990s, and the technology is manufactured by Accuray, Inc of Sunnyvale, California. While FDA-approved, the Cyberknife® protocol is still considered investigational, with few published studies to date and limited availability. At Stanford, Accuray's Cyberknife® is now being combined with Varian Medical Systems' IG-IMRT technology.

I have reservations about the the Cyberknife® based on its very penetrating radiation dose. The bottom line is that whenever you hypofractionate radiation (fewer treatments over a shorter time frame using higher radiation doses per treatment), you are making a compromise for the long haul. That is, expect significantly increased side effects over time. With prostate treatment, we're talking about progressive damage to the bladder, urethra, rectum, neurovascular bundles, etc. over time. These symptoms will most likely begin to manifest between beyond 12 months after treatment. I would never consider utilizing this type of modality at our center unless a patient's life expectancy is 6 months or less. The significance of fractionated versus continuous radiation delivery will be discussed further in the pages ahead.

"Why Would Anyone Choose Cyberknife?" This is the title of an entry on the Prostate Cancer Blog, posted in May 2007 by Dr. Louis Potters, founder of the New York Prostate Institute. Dr. Potters quotes an article in the International *Journal of Radiation Oncology, Biology and Physics* (vol. 67, No. 4, pp 1099) in which the author B.L. Madsen, M.D. writes," … in a Phase I/II trial of SHARP (Stereotactic Hypofractionated Accurate Radiotherapy for localize prostate cancer) the actuarial 48-month biochemical freedom from relapse is 70% using the ASTRO definition."

Dr. Potters and many others know that these results are not nearly as good as the results widely reported with IMRT and seeds—with long-term (14 years and more) data at the Dattoli Center Center. Without mincing words and pitting noted researchers against one another, the biggest obstacle facing Cyberknife® (or Gammaknife or SHARP or any other such stereotactic hypofractionated therapy) for prostate cancer treatment is the lack of published clinical data to prove that it provides any better results than currently proven therapies. So why would anyone choose it?

Facilities and physicians promoting Cyberknife® have big investments to recoup. The marketing machines are grinding out stories and material to glorify their products. "Cyber" is a sexy word in advertising buzz today. And, while the therapy has been successfully used with treating intracranial tumors for years, its application for soft tissue tumors (such as prostate) is glorified as "new"—as if everything "new" is "better."

Website material from Accuray (manufacturer of the Cyberknife®) touts its ability for clinical flexibility, delineation of tumor versus normal tissue for targeting, shorter treatment time and relatively low toxicity of the rectum and bladder.

But beware. A physician at a large CK facility in Oklahoma (who has threatened us not to use his name), in an Internet patient support forum admits that "generally speaking, failure (at least in our hands) occurs most often when all our imaging does not make it possible to determine where the tumor stops and the normal tissue starts. We usually err on the side of including more volume, but sometimes we just can't make the correct decision. We have sometimes been able to go back and re-treat the area we missed."

As I will discuss in greater detail below, the primary goal of combination therapy (4D IG-IMRT and seeds) at the Dattoli Cancer Center is to stop the identified tumor in its tracks, but the larger ultimate goal is to treat the entire gland. We know that whatever biochemical forces were in place to cause the growth of the primary tumor are at work, albeit at a slower pace, throughout the gland. All the intense focal efforts to treat only the tumor is leaving the rest of the gland untouched–and ripe for future cancer growth.

With 4D IG-IMRT and DART and subsequent Palladium-103 brachytherapy, we are able to sculpt the radiation dose to surround the gland and spare the central core housing the urethra – attacking the active tumor cells and rendering the remainder of gland fallow for future tumor growth. It is our goal to have prostate cancer be a one-time event in the man's life.

Cyberknife® proponents herald their 5-day treatment vs the 23-day 4D IG-IMRT program, as "more convenient" for the patient. How "convenient", we ask, will it be for the patient to face a repeat performance 3, 4, 8 or more years down the road? Or how convenient will it be in the long run (late effects of radiation) when patients develop urethral and/or rectal fistulas, bladder damage, rectal ulcerations or perforations requiring colostomies, hip and bone necrosis–which are all documented complications from hypofractionated radiation?

What is Brachytherapy?

Brachytherapy, also called *interstitial implantation therapy,* involves the placement of tiny radioactive seeds or pellets directly into the prostate gland. The radioactive seeds can either be inserted temporarily, or can remain permanently in place within the prostate. They provide a high dose of radiation that is concentrated in the prostate. Permanent seeds pose no health threat to the patient, as they decay within 6 months to a year, and thereafter, they become inert.

Brachytherapy has a fairly long history. As early as 1917, a crude form of seed implantation using radium needles was performed at what is now Memorial Sloan-Kettering Cancer Center. The chief of urology at that time, Dr. Barringer, was so enthusiastic about the procedure that he concluded his report in the *Journal of the American Medical Association,* "…because of the initial success of radium treatment, I now take the stand that no patient with prostate cancer should be operated on." In fact, the technology had not yet been developed that would make the procedure effective. The 1980s saw renewed interest in seed implants because the development of ultrasound imaging, CT scans and fluoroscopic techniques allowed for precise planning and monitoring of where the seeds should be placed. Since that time, brachytherapy has become a standard, mainstream treatment for prostate cancer that is widely available throughout the U.S.

As with external radiation therapy, a number of technical refinements in the seed implant procedure have led to improved results and increasing popularity. In the old days (as recently as the 1970s), seed implants required major abdominal surgery. Seeds of radioactive isotopes were manually implanted into the prostate using needles, but the procedure was essentially carried out blind and achieved poor results because of a lack of precision in placing the seeds. Poor placement led to "cold" spots within the prostate gland that did not receive a sufficient dose of radiation to destroy the cancer.

In more recent years, a minimally invasive technique has been devised for implanting the seeds in the prostate without open surgery (known as "transperineal implantation"). Guided by ultrasound and fluoroscopy, the seeds are dispensed through tiny hollow needles which are inserted through the perineum (the area between the scrotum and anus). A template or grid is used to precisely guide the placement of the needles. Ultrasound allows for real time imaging and dynamic visualization. As the technology has evolved with color-flow Doppler ultrasound, a more precise, three-dimensional image of the prostate can be generated, and the seeds can be more accurately placed, where they will be most effective (See Color Inset Images 2-A, 2-B, 2-C, 2-D, 2-E, 2F). As with external radiation therapy, the strategy has been to target and destroy the cancer with minimal exposure to surrounding healthy tissue and organs. The computerized guidance system helps determine where the seeds should go, how deeply they should be inserted, and how strong their radiation should be. At our institution, we use both pre-planning and intraoperative dosimetry for optimal seed placement.

Brachytherapy with ultrasound and fluoroscopic guidance has a number of advantages over conventional external beam radiation therapy. The standard dose of radiation used with EBRT is approximately 7000 cGy, calculated to be the highest dose which is safe and well tolerated by the patient. By contrast, seed implants are placed internally to deliver radiation directly to the prostate while sparing surrounding organs. As a consequence, higher doses of radiation (exceeding 12,000 cGy) can be administered to the area of the prostate, while tumorous sites often receive doses in excess of 20,000 cGy. In addition, the radiation delivered by seeds is continuous over the time they are active, working around the clock to kill the cancer. By contrast, all other forms of radiation, including HDR (see below) are fractionated, which means the radiation is administered only in intermittent doses.

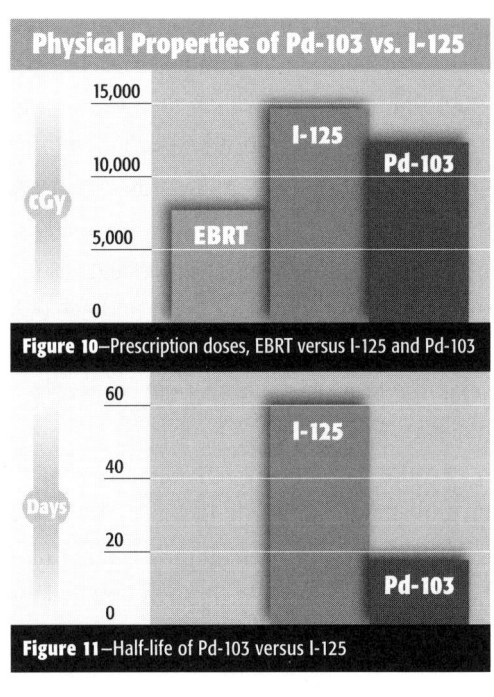

Figure 10–Prescription doses, EBRT versus I-125 and Pd-103

Figure 11–Half-life of Pd-103 versus I-125

A number of radiation sources have been used for interstitial implantation. The most commonly used permanent implants are encapsulated isotopes of either Palladium-103 or Iodine-125. Pd-103 has a significantly shorter half-life (the period of time until its output of radiation is halved) and a greater initial radiation dose than I-125 (see Figures 10-11). With palladium, the radiation dosage is delivered in three to four months compared to up to one year with iodine. Because the radiation is active for a shorter period with palladium, temporary side effects such as urinary distress are shorter in duration.

A new implant isotope, Cesium-131, is currently being investigated. It has a shorter half life (9.7 days) and a higher average energy (29 KeV) than both Iodine-125 and Palladium-103. This means that Cesium-131 is likely to deliver a higher dose to surrounding tissue over a shorter period of time, and therefore, may increase the risk of complications. Dose response data using this isotope will take many years of further study.

What is High Does Rate (HDR) Brachytherapy?

High Dose Rate brachytherapy refers to temporary implants that utilize Iridium-192. This form of therapy is not new. It was first utilized in the early 1960s at Memorial Sloan-Kettering Cancer Center and has remained essentially unchanged since that time, with the exception of the current use of microprocessors and advanced imaging techniques.

The Iridium-192 isotope is encased inside a hollow plastic catheter less than 2 millimeters in diameter. Typically guided by ultrasound, these implants are inserted into the prostate and then removed, with two to four separate procedures spread over two to three days. HDR sources deliver much higher doses of radiation in a much shorter period of time than permanent implants.

MODALITY	TYPICAL DOSE	DELIVERY
3D-CRT	7000–8000 cGy	Fractionated
IMRT	7000–9000 cGy	Fractionated
Protons/Neutrons	7000–8000 cGy	Fractionated
Pd-103/I-125 Brachytherapy (Monotherapy)	12,500/14,400 cGy	Continuous
HDR Ir-192 (Monotherapy)	?	Fractionated
3D-CRT/IMRT and Pd-103/I-125	4000–5000 cGy 8000–12,000 cGy	Fractionated Continuous
EBRT and HDR Ir-192	4000–5000 cGy 1500–2500 cGy	Fractionated Fractionated

A Comparison of Radiotherapy Modalities for Treatment of Localized (loco-regional) Prostate Cancer. Continuous versus Fractionated Radiation Therapies.

Some limited studies have reported cure rates with the temporary HDR procedure that are comparable to those achieved by permanent implants. There is, however, less data regarding outcomes and side effects when compared to permanent implants. The HDR approach is not widely used for reasons of convenience and practicality. If performed in one session, the patient *must* remain in a semi-lithotomy position (legs pulled up) for upwards of 72 hours, with needles remaining in the prostate throughout this duration.

Like external beam radiation, HDR is a form of fractionated high dose rate photon radiation, which may increase the risk of damaging side effects in the long run to the urethra, rectum and bladder. Temporary implants usually require hospitalization and repeated implant procedures as opposed to the single permanent implant technique which can be done essentially on an out-patient basis. There may also be a greater risk of complications with HDR because of the extremely penetrating, high dose of radiation delivered by the Iridium-192 isotope (1000 to 2000 cGy in a matter of minutes to the entire body). The risk of complications is likely to be increased when fewer fractions (fewer treatment sessions) are utilized, since patients are being exposed to higher doses of radiation albeit for shorter periods of time. In the past, when at the request of some patients, I performed HDR brachytherapy, I used a minimum of five fractions, in order to try to ensure greater safety. But today, when HDR brachytherapists routinely use only two or three fractions, there is considerable cause for concern about morbidity in the long term. The discussion that follows will be devoted to permanent Pd-103 and I-125 implantation.

How are Permanent Seed Implants Planned and Performed?

At our institution, patients routinely undergo a pre-treatment staging and planning color-flow Doppler ultrasound. That test, coupled with other staging studies (e.g., EMRI, MRSI or dynamic MRI, ProstaScint® and 18F-FDG Fluoride PET/CT Fusion) will allow us to visualize various physical aspects of the gland, such as its size, shape, and contour. These tests also provide detailed information about the volume and location of the tumor (or tumors). With that information, we are able to determine exactly where the seeds should be placed. Additionally, this pre-treatment analysis may tell

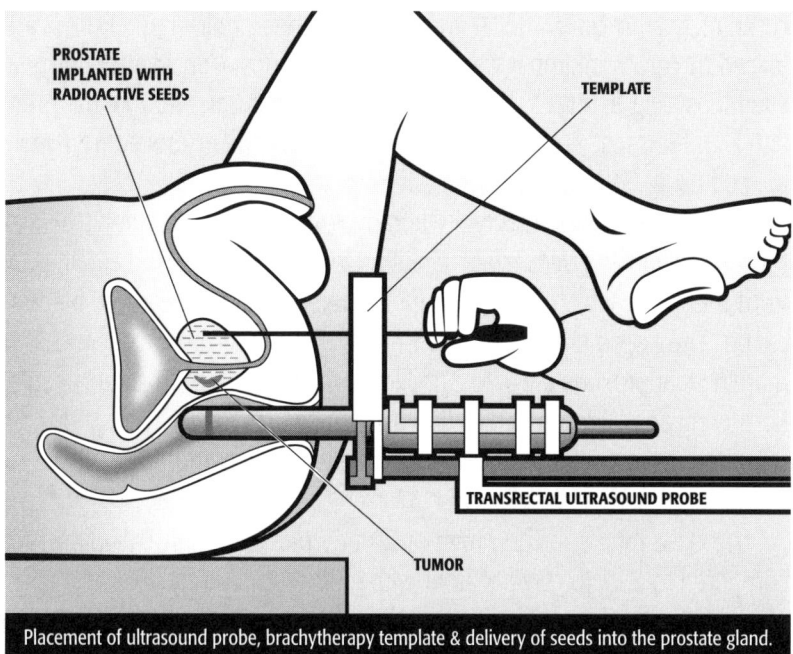

PROSTATE
IMPLANTED WITH
RADIOACTIVE SEEDS

TEMPLATE

TRANSRECTAL ULTRASOUND PROBE

TUMOR

Placement of ultrasound probe, brachytherapy template & delivery of seeds into the prostate gland.

us if the pubic bones are going pose any sort of obstacle when we perform the procedure. This is known as pubic arch interference, which we can usually circumvent by positioning the patient more advantageously. Later, in the operating room, the original plan will be modified since the gland position or contour changes when the pelvic muscles are relaxed under anesthesia. This is referred to as real time intraoperative planning to achieve optimal dosimetry.

Prior to the implant procedure, I ask my patients not to eat after midnight the night before and the morning of the implant. A patient is admitted to the hospital as an outpatient for 23-hour observation. After admission, he is routinely given a prophylactic antibiotic. The patient is then brought into a dedicated brachytherapy surgical suite, and there undergoes an antisceptic skin cleansing. That is usually a Betadine solution applied to the perineal region. We also provide him with pre-implant bowel cleansing instructions and are ready to proceed with the procedure after administering a local anesthetic (in most cases epidural or spinal anesthesia).

The procedure is done with the patient lying on his back, with his legs pulled up in what is called the *extended lithotomy position.* His legs are completely limp since a local anesthesia has been delivered. His feet are placed in comfortable booties and held in stirrups. Considerable time is spent ensuring that the patient is in the proper position and that the prostate is in the most desirable position. Then the implant procedure is performed using both ultrasound and fluoroscopic guidance.

The isotopes used for brachytherapy (except for Ir-192) don't deliver much radiation at a distance of a centimeter or centimeter and a half away from the gland, which is, for example, where the rectum and the bladder reside. The seeds are placed precisely at the site of the cancer within a margin of approximately 1 to 5 millimeters outside the prostate capsule. By this means, aided by color-flow Doppler ultrasound visualization, we can often deliver two to five times the dose with brachytherapy that we can with any other kind of radiation.

The dose rate is in the range of 20 cGy per hour with Palladium-103 compared to 5 to 10 cGy per hour with Iodine-125. A total dose of 12,500 cGy is typically delivered with Palladium-103 to full decay, while 14,400 cGy is typically delivered with Iodine-125. If I am supplementing the seed implant by preceding it with IMRT, then I have to reduce the dose of the implant. With this combined or integrated approach, patients typically receive 4500 cGy of external radiation to a limited pelvic field, followed approximately three to six weeks later by a Palladium-103 "boost." When combined with IMRT, the prescribed minimum Pd-103 dose to the prostate is 8000 to 9000 cGy, with a suitable margin.

Seed implants are performed in a specially designed operating room (OR) where computers are accessible for intra-operative modifications. A well-trained OR staff is utilized for the procedure. Local anesthesia (spinal versus epidural) is preferred. The advantage of a local anesthetic is that the patient feels little or no discomfort upon awakening, including that of a catheter, which is put into place during the implant procedure. Anti-inflammatory medications and antibiotics are routinely administered during and after the procedure (intraoperative and postoperative).

We maintain computers in the operating room since the contour of the prostate gland typically changes. This is an extremely common occurrence since this is the first time we are looking at the prostate in a relaxed position without the pelvic muscles surrounding it being very tense. Because the pa-

STATE OF THE ART
BRACHYTHERAPY
AND IMRT

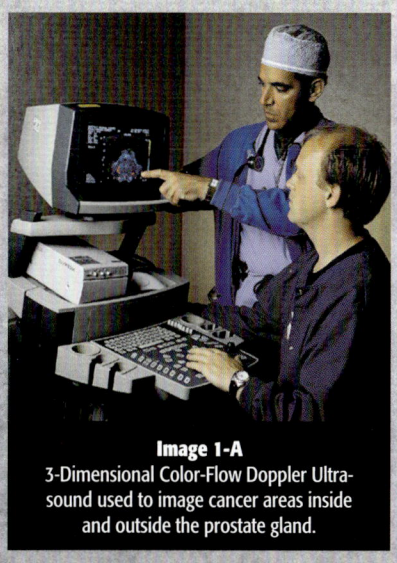

Image 1-A
3-Dimensional Color-Flow Doppler Ultrasound used to image cancer areas inside and outside the prostate gland.

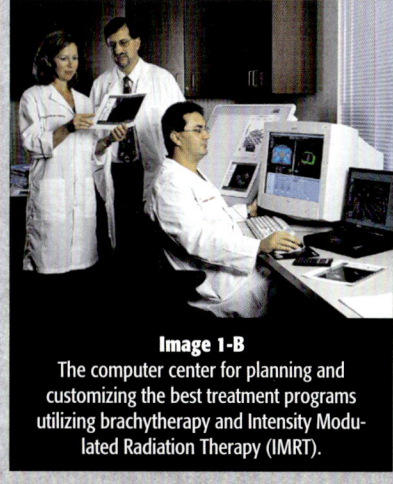

Image 1-B
The computer center for planning and customizing the best treatment programs utilizing brachytherapy and Intensity Modulated Radiation Therapy (IMRT).

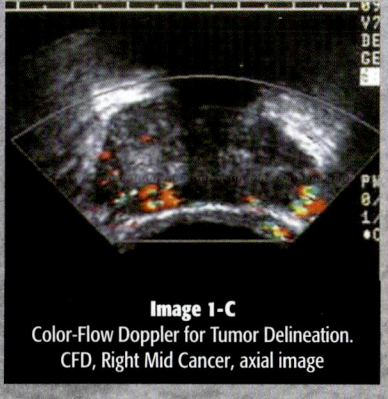

Image 1-C
Color-Flow Doppler for Tumor Delineation. CFD, Right Mid Cancer, axial image

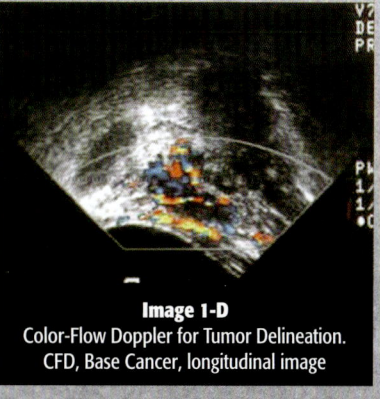

Image 1-D
Color-Flow Doppler for Tumor Delineation. CFD, Base Cancer, longitudinal image

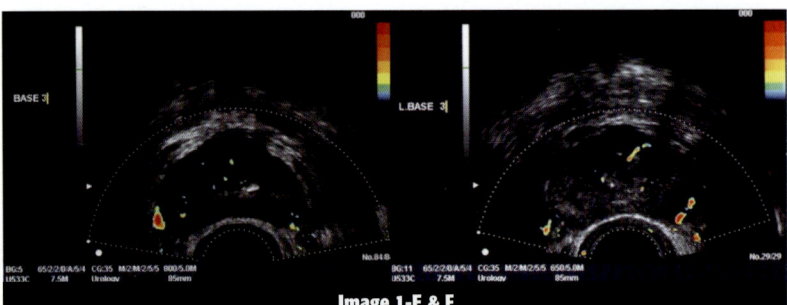

Image 1-E & F
3-Dimensional Color-Flow Doppler Ultrasound Images showing blood perfusion (hypervascularity) in the vicinity of tumor sites.

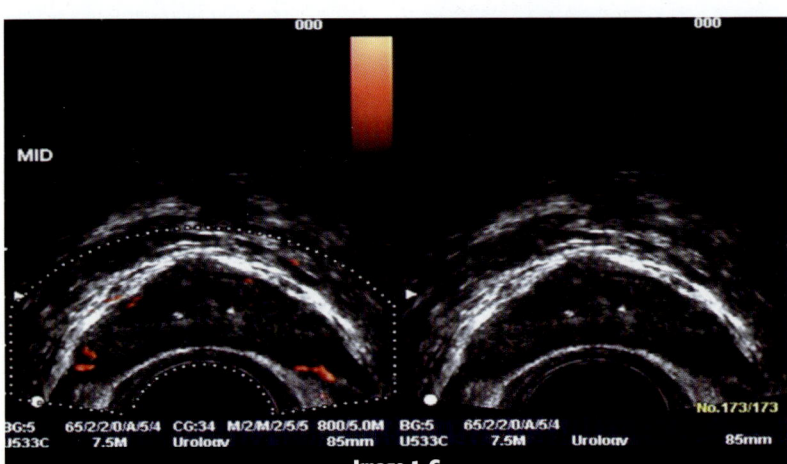

Image 1-G
Comparison of Color-Flow Doppler image (left) with conventional gray-scale ultrasound image (right) of the same patient. Note: The bright red areas in the Color-Flow Doppler image reveal the location of suspected cancer sites, which are not visible using gray-scale ultrasound imaging.

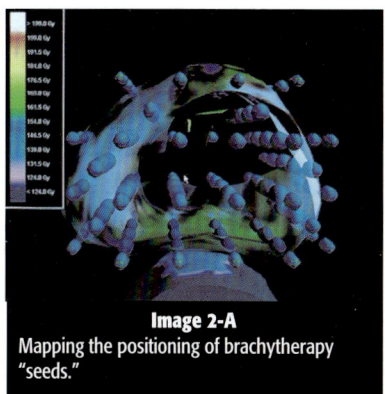

Image 2-A
Mapping the positioning of brachytherapy "seeds."

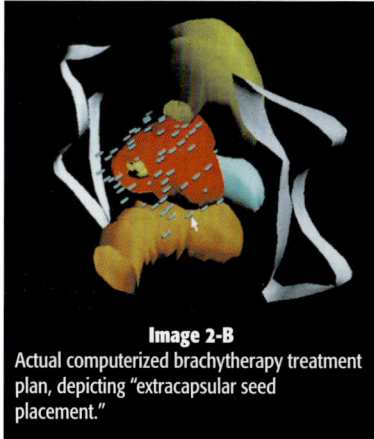

Image 2-B
Actual computerized brachytherapy treatment plan, depicting "extracapsular seed placement."

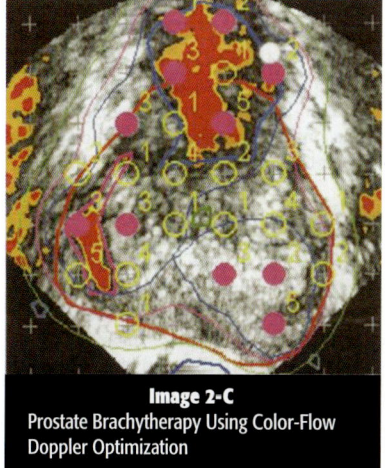

Image 2-C
Prostate Brachytherapy Using Color-Flow Doppler Optimization

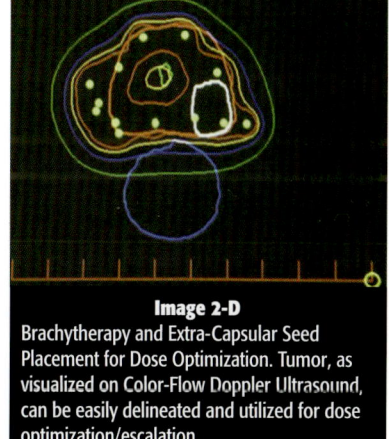

Image 2-D
Brachytherapy and Extra-Capsular Seed Placement for Dose Optimization. Tumor, as visualized on Color-Flow Doppler Ultrasound, can be easily delineated and utilized for dose optimization/escalation.

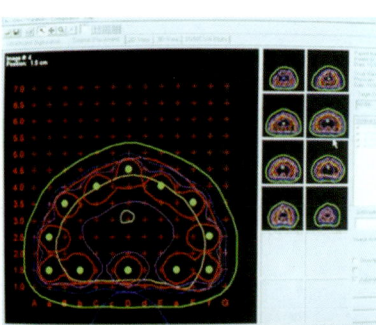

Image 2-E
Brachytherapy Dose Optimization Using Extra-Capsular Seeds. Tumor, as visualized on Color-Flow Doppler Ultrasound, can be easily delineated and utilized for dose optimization/escalation.

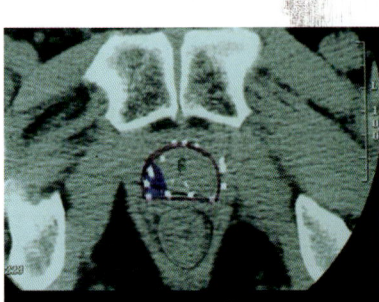

Image 2-F
Brachytherapy Dose Optimization. Tumor delineation on post-implant CT for dosimetric analysis.

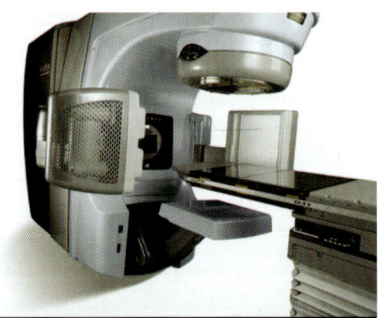

Image 6
A linear accelerator for delivering 4D IG-IMRT, complete with on-board imaging capabilities and the 'exact couch' system.

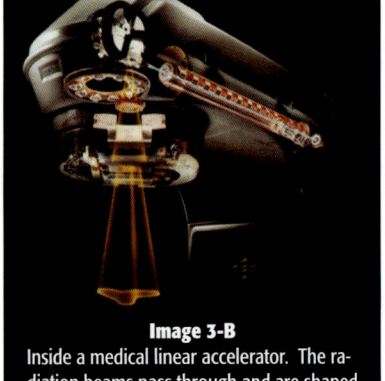

Image 3-B
Inside a medical linear accelerator. The radiation beams pass through and are shaped by a device called a multileaf collimator so that it conforms to the shape of the tumor. Courtesy of Varian Medical Systems.

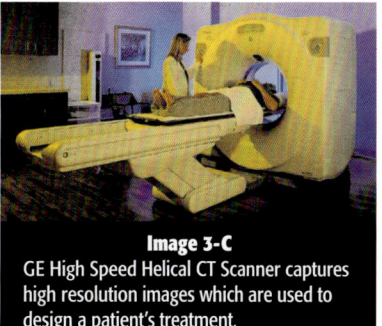

Image 3-C
GE High Speed Helical CT Scanner captures high resolution images which are used to design a patient's treatment.

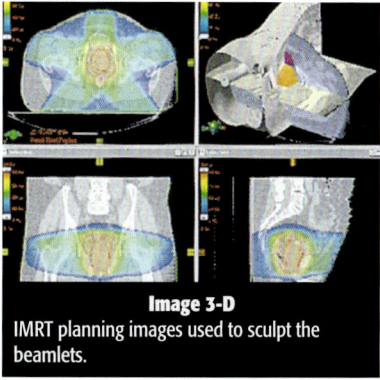

Image 3-D
IMRT planning images used to sculpt the beamlets.

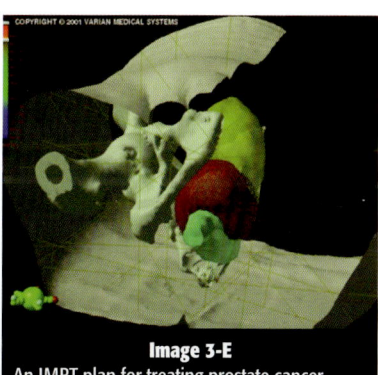

Image 3-E
An IMRT plan for treating prostate cancer, concentrating the radiation dose in the tumor (red) while avoiding the nearby bladder (yellow) and rectum (green). Courtesy of Varian Medical Systems.

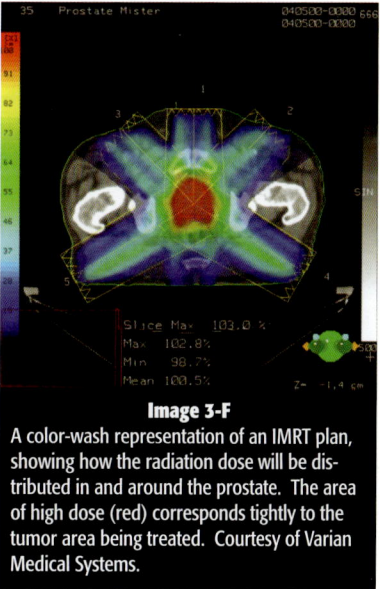

Image 3-F
A color-wash representation of an IMRT plan, showing how the radiation dose will be distributed in and around the prostate. The area of high dose (red) corresponds tightly to the tumor area being treated. Courtesy of Varian Medical Systems.

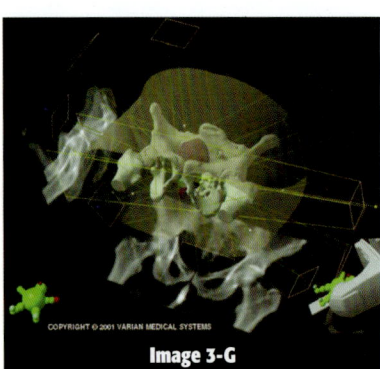

Image 3-G
An IMRT beam arrangement for treating prostate cancer, viewed in three dimensions. Courtesy of Varian Medical Systems.

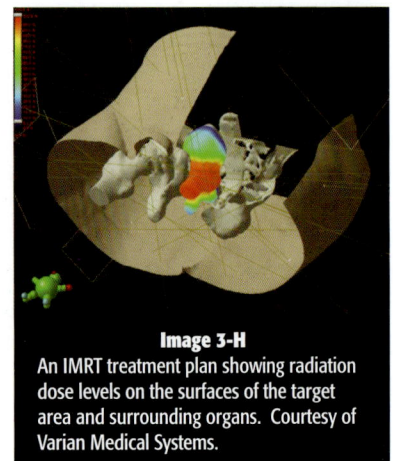

Image 3-H
An IMRT treatment plan showing radiation dose levels on the surfaces of the target area and surrounding organs. Courtesy of Varian Medical Systems.

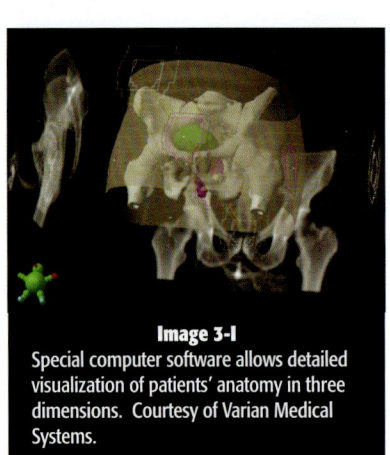

Image 3-I
Special computer software allows detailed visualization of patients' anatomy in three dimensions. Courtesy of Varian Medical Systems.

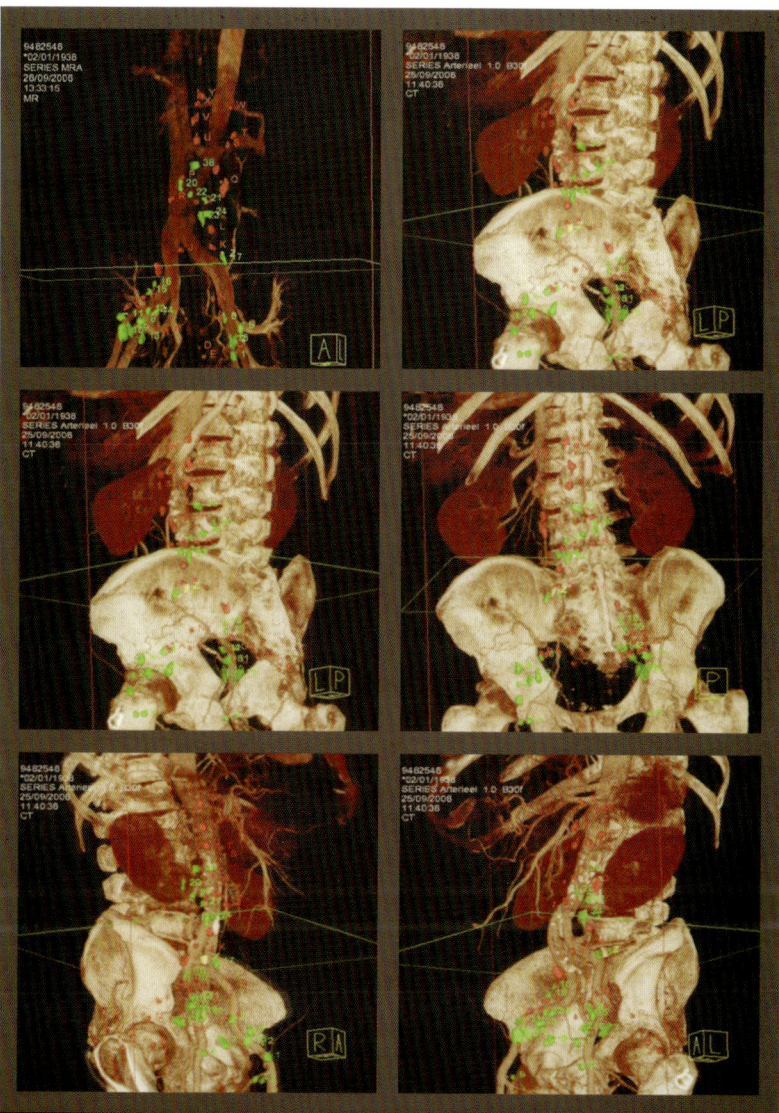

Image 3-J
The Combidex® imaging technique allows us to clearly distinguish between benign and malignant lymph nodes and to construct 3-dimensional maps to guide clinicians. Combidex® is a nano-particle test that utilizes ferrous oxide (Ferumoxtran-10) as a contrast agent. The patient is scanned after infusion. This test is currently awaiting FDA approval, and in the meantime some patients travel to the Netherlands to undergo testing. Fused with MRI, Combidex® has opened up whole new areas that we can treat. In practice, the predictive accuracy approaches 100% and it can pick up metastases as small as 1 millimeter in size.

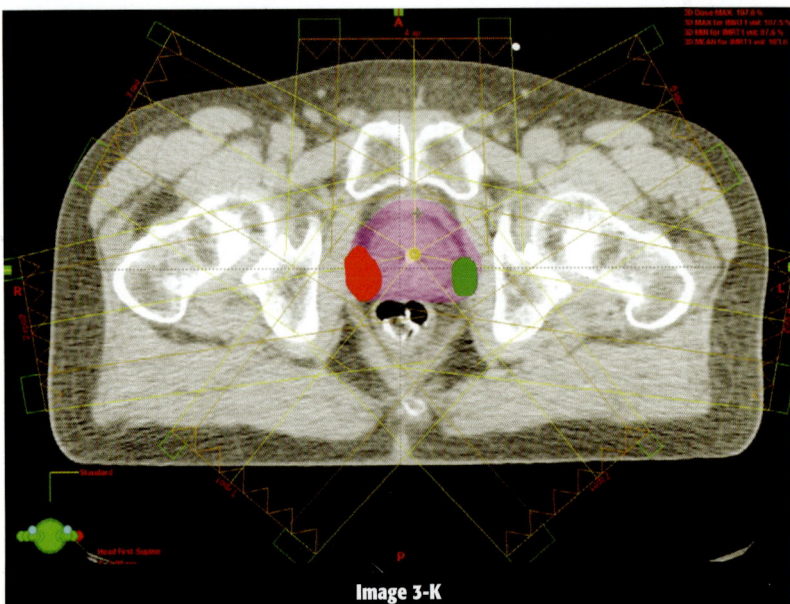

Image 3-K

The first treatment plan that is produced from the simulation CT scan is called IMRT1, with 7 fields placed in the pattern. The purple area is the volume of interest, which includes the prostate and seminal vesicles.

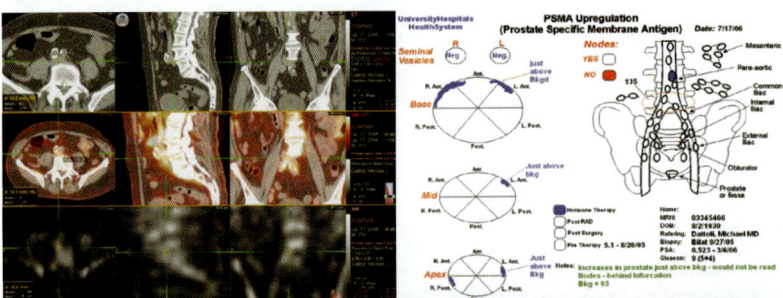

Image 3-L

ProstaScint® is another diagnostic test that enables doctors to determine lymph node involvement. ProstaScint® can be fused with helical CT or with MRI or with CT/PET scans. A pictorial analysis for this patient appears to the right of the scanned images.

tient has undergone a local anesthetic, he cannot tense up around the ultrasound probe which is placed in the rectum. Intraoperative modifications of the plan are made as necessary. Seed migration is not a problem since I use a special seed with very concave ends, and the tissue lodges in the edges, anchoring the seeds in place. I only use "free seeds" (rather than "stranded seeds") because this allows me maximal flexibility to make intraoperative changes as indicated and also allows me to place seeds in extracapsular locations. The tumor dose is escalated by locating it with color-flow Doppler ultrasound and by using seeds of different strengths to dose escalate the tumor and to dose demodulate critical structures such as the urethra, bladder and rectum.

The actual procedure, that is, the placement of the needles and insertion of the seeds, rarely takes longer than twenty-five minutes. The set-up time and preparation of the patient may take longer, and therefore, I generally book an hour and a half in the OR, because the patient has to be placed in the proper position and prepped for the procedure. It's very important to have the patient in a position that is identical to that of his pre-planning study in an attempt to duplicate the initial plan. In practice, the pre-plan enables the dosimetrist to know how many seeds to order, though the plan will typically change with the use of real time intraoperative optimization methods. When performing the procedure, special crisscross anchoring needles are used to maximally immobilize the prostate gland. These two crisscross needles are inserted transperineally, obliquely into the prostate, using finger and fluoroscopic guidance. These needles are left in place during the procedure to anchor the prostate in place.

Seeds are commonly placed in extracapsular positions to further target the tumor, which may be microscopically escaping from the gland. The technique of placing seeds 1 to 5 millimeters outside the gland also allows for reduction of the urethral dose. This is important since the main side effect of brachytherapy is temporary urethritis. Additionally, we have reported this technique allows for treating patients who have had prior TURPS with a far reduced incontinence rate.

After the procedure, the patient is transferred to a private room and monitored closely throughout his stay. Although many brachytherapists discharge their patients soon after the implant is complete, I prefer to keep the patient overnight. The indwelling catheter is left in place for a minimum of 12 hours and dislodges any tissue, clots or debris that could present future problems (urinary blockage). The catheter is removed only when upon inspection the urine is perfectly clear. Usually, I keep the catheters in until two o'clock in the morning. That saves a lot of grief for both the patient and for me by eliminating those calls that I might receive at 2:00 A.M. when the patient potentially has some blockage. By keeping the catheter in and irrigating the bladder, we have eliminated this problem.

For the most part, patients have a very easy time with seed implants. The most common question asked after the procedure is, "When are you going to start?" Many are still waiting for the procedure to begin when they realize it has already taken place. Patients rarely complain of specific pains in the perineal region, that area where the seeds are implanted between the scrotal sac and the anus. The only discomfort that a patient may have is more likely to be a consequence of the catheter later in the day or evening when the regional anesthetic has worn off. That may be felt more than the tiny needles which are utilized to insert the seeds.

The patient is discharged the morning following the procedure, usually in excellent spirits and ready to return home whether far away or locally. He must first report to our center. Prior to his leaving here, special stereo-shift x-rays and helical CT scans are taken to count seeds and to ensure there are no potential complications (for example, absess formation or hematomas from bleeding, though these are uncommon). Patients will then return for a comprehensive evaluation at approximately 3 months, and then 6 to 12 months thereafter. Ultimately, I request that my patients return annually.

Which Patients are Eligible for Brachytherapy?

Most patients can safely tolerate the implant procedure as it is minimally invasive and requires only light anesthesia. Men with a history of heart disease or stroke are usually given a thorough medical evaluation, including a cardiac stress test, before proceeding with seed implantation.

If you are a candidate for surgery, you are almost surely also a candidate for seed implants, as both treatments are most effective with early stage cancers. In addition, many men who would not be candidates for surgery—

those patients over the age of 70, or those men with other health conditions that rule out major surgery—may qualify as candidates for seeding, which is obviously a much less invasive procedure than radical prostatectomy.

The most important factor in determining a patient's eligibility for seeding is how far the cancer has spread. If the cancer is localized, that is, confined to the prostate gland, then it is more likely to be curable, with either surgery or seeding. Once the cancer has spread beyond the prostate capsule, it is not curable by implantation alone, because the seed implants do not radiate enough area around the prostate to destroy any cancer that may have spread beyond the prostate capsule. These patients are similarly not candidates for radical prostatectomy.

Patients with stage T1 are most likely to have cancer that is confined to the prostate, and therefore, curable with seed implantation alone. With that said, having treated over the years thousands of low risk patients with seeds alone, and followed them for 10 to 20 years, I have witnessed an increased failure rate (as many as 50% of these patients typically after 10 years) when compared to low risk or even intermediate risk patients who were treated with a combination of seeds and external beam radiation. For this reason, I encourage combined treatment even for low risk patients since the side effect profile is the same or even slightly reduced with the combined approach. The last telephone call I ever want to make to a patient is to tell him that his PSA is rising. I believe the multi-modality approach improves survival rates. By combining seeds and external beam radiation, the cancer is being exposed to two different forms of radiation and is more likely to be eradicated.

Patients with locally advanced disease may be treated either with external radiation or with a combination of seed implants and external radiation (preferably IMRT). These patients include those with one or more of the following risk factors: stage equal to or greater than T2b, a Gleason score greater than or equal to 7, a PSA greater than 10, an elevated PAP, an adverse immunohistochemical marker, perineural invasion (PNI), or radiographic evidence of extracapsular extension (as indicated by color-flow Doppler ultrasound or endorectal MRI, MRSI or dynamic MRI, ProstaScint®/CT Fusion, 18F-FDG Fluoride PET/CT Fusion, and other advanced imaging techniques).

Seed implants should only be considered by patients who are young enough and healthy enough to live long enough to benefit from being cured. Excellent candidates are men from their forties to their seventies, with localized prostate cancer. As mentioned earlier, some men in their eighties who are in good health may also benefit from implantation, and an increasing number of men in their thirties are now being treated with these methods. After all, younger patients stand to benefit most from therapies that will preserve their quality of life, including continence and erectile function.

Patients who have had a portion of their prostate removed with a previous TURP may be at increased risk for urinary incontinence after seeding, in which case, special modifications of seed placement may be necessary when possible (peripheral seed loading and especially sparing the external sphincter). Patients with enlarged prostates and those men who have difficulty with urination prior to treatment may have more severe urinary problems after implantation. Treatment is typically limited to men with prostates less than 60 cubic centimeters volume. For patients with enlarged prostates, two or three months of hormonal therapy before implantation may be prescribed in order to shrink the gland. Larger glands may be implanted based on anatomical considerations.

What are the Most Common Myths About Brachytherapy and IMRT?

Myth # 1

"Your tumor is too aggressive to be effectively treated by brachytherapy." This assertion is often made by urologists, who suggest that a high PSA and/ or a high Gleason score disqualifies patients for seed implants. In fact, the published results of brachytherapy with intermediate and high risk patients are superior to surgical results even at the leading surgical centers.

Myth # 2

"Your prostate gland is too small for brachytherapy." Patients with smaller glands may hear this from their urologists, but the statement is absolutely false. Brachytherapy can treat smaller glands very effectively, specifically, by putting seeds outside the prostate capsule (the technique known as "extracapsular seed placement"). By placing the seeds in this fashion, the dose to the urethra can actually be decreased while the target area receives an effective, cancercidal dose.

Myth # 3

"Your prostate gland is too large for brachytherapy." This is another urological myth. By extending the lithotomy position, which is the position with the legs up in the air, and/or by using steering needles, problems with pubic arch interference can be circumvented. In this way, seed implants can be utilized with patients who have larger prostates. In addition, larger glands can often be downsized with hormonal therapy.

Myth # 4

"Once you've had brachytherapy, you've burned your bridges. Surgery cannot be performed after implantation, and you won't have any other salvage options if the seeds fail." In fact, an expert surgeon will be able to remove the prostate after seed implantation. However, the patient may and probably would choose one of a number of other options. Since he chose not to have surgery in the first place, he may choose re-seeding, with or without 4-Dimensional Image Guided IMRT. At the Dattoli Cancer Center, another isotope will be used, because clearly if the cancer failed the first isotope, doctors want to give it something else that it's not ac-climated to. So if a patient was seeded with Iodine-125, he may have an improved outcome with Palladium-103. The patient can also choose cryo-surgery as a salvage therapy, or biothermy, which combines cryosurgery and hyperthermia. High Intensity Frequency Ultrasound would be another option, and researchers are working on vaccines for which there are clini-cal trials underway.

Myth # 5

"You are a young patient, and therefore, radiation may increase your risk of developing a secondary cancer." There is a great deal of data show-ing this assertion to be false. Recent studies have reported that contempo-rary radiation does not increase the risk of future colo-rectal cancer (Ken-dall, et al, *Int. J Rad Onc,* Vol 65, No 3, 2006, and Gotman, et al, *Int. J Rad Onc,* Vol 66, No 1, 2006). This myth is based on old data when radiation oncologists were treating with external beams and large-field boxes, and they were basically treating normal tissue in addition to the prostate or lymph nodes in order to deliver radiation to those structures. The accuracy of the current state-of-the-art technology eliminates the risk of developing secondary cancers after brachytherapy and 4D IG-IMRT.

Myth # 6

"You are too young to have brachytherapy. Younger patients have radical surgery; older patients get radiation therapy." This is yet another falsehood. In this regard, outstanding biochemical outcomes have been reported for younger patients and this group has the most to gain (reduced risk of urinary incontinence and/or erectile dysfunction). Of the numerous studies published by Blasko (2005), Kwok (2002), Kollmeir (2003), Dattoli (2007), all have mean and median follow-up which is equal to or longer than the surgical series published in the PSA era.

Myth # 7

"You are too old to have brachytherapy." The truth is that older patients tolerate brachytherapy as well as younger patients. Many patients as well as doctors are not aware of the fact that life expectancy is quite long and becoming longer with each passing year (see discussion, pp. 14-17). As such, more and more older patients can and should be treated, especially with non-invasive treatments such as brachytherapy and other sophisticated forms of radiation.

Myth # 8

"If you had a prior TURP (transurethral resection of the prostate), you are not a candidate for brachytherapy." Many urologists suggest that a prior TURP is a contraindication for seed implants, but that is simply not the case. The Dattoli team has published extensively on this subject, showing that it can be done, but the patient with a prior TURP must be carefully evaluated. Each patient is different. There has to be enough tissue to put the seeds into the gland. If the TURP was a "Roto-Rooter" and removed too much tissue, there may not be enough tissue left to anchor the seeds. In addition, special efforts must be made to avoid incontinence. Another issue is avoiding a hot apex, which is the bottom of the gland. A patient who has had a TURP has already had his internal sphincter removed, and so we have to be concerned about his external sphincter, his lower sphincter. We have learned that external radiation (4D IG-IMRT), combined with brachytherapy, reduces the risk of problems with these patients (see "How are Implants Modified for Patients with Prior TURPs?").

With regard to this issue, please note: Modern peripheral seed placement where epithelial (TURP) defect is limited to ≤110% of the minimum peripheral dose, results in reduced incontinence/leakage are similar to that of non-TURP patients, taking into account the following considerations:

➤ The gland must have sufficient tissue remaining to anchor seeds.

➤ Case selection is paramount to avoid overly extensive TURP.

➤ Avoidance of hot apex and supplemental IMRT may even further reduce risks of urinary incontinence/leakage.

Myth # 9

"You are too overweight to have brachytherapy." Contrary to this notion, the reality is that brachytherapy patients who are overweight enjoy a higher rate of success with seed implants than with surgery. In fact, brachytherapy is the most preferred treatment for obese patients. A high body mass index (BMI) translates into increased hospital stays after surgery. Comparing surgery and brachytherapy in terms of biochemical failure with high BMI patients, as the body mass index goes up, the surgical relapse rate goes up as well, while brachytherapy achieves excellent results with these patients.

Myth # 10

"You have an elevated AUA score and that precludes you from having brachytherapy." The AUA score provides a profile of urinary and rectal symptoms. An elevated AUA score in many cases is not a contraindication for seed implants. Even patients with voiding symptoms can tolerate brachytherapy. This may be because doctors have learned how to micromanage these symptoms. There have been a number of studies investigating long term urinary morbidity after seed implantation. One study demonstrated that "patients who presented with marked urinary symptoms prior to brachytherapy had the most significant improvement in symptoms and quality of life after brachytherapy at a median follow-up of 31 months" (Stone et al, *J. Brachy. Int.*, Vol 2, 2003). Another recent study showed there was no significant difference in the overall long-term urinary and quality of life (QOL) scores when brachytherapy patients were compared to a control group (Merrick et al, *IJROBP,* Vol 56, 2003).

When is Hormonal Therapy Used Prior to Brachytherapy?

Hormonal treatment is typically optional for patients having intermediate risk features but encouraged for patients having high risk features. With the low-risk or mildly aggressive cancers, unless the size of the gland is markedly large, we don't normally give the conventional hormonal therapy (combined hormonal blockade using an anti-androgen and an LHRH agonist, such as Lupron®, Eligard®, Zoladex® or TRELSTAR®), since this form of therapy may result in untoward side effects such as impotence, hot flashes and potential weakness. We often prescribe a milder, modified version of hormones (e.g., oral anti-androgens, such as Eulexin® or Casodex®), something that is just enough to arrest the cancer and allow the patient to make a more relaxed decision about treatment, without the rush or urgency that are often associated with it (see Chapter Eight: Treating Metastatic Disease).

Why are More Patients Choosing to Combine Seed Implants with IMRT?

Over the past decade I have seen the pendulum swing dramatically from patients in the past who strongly desired to undergo seed implantations alone to more recent patients who desire the combination method of IMRT and brachytherapy. This trend is probably due to a number of factors. These days many patients do extensive research and find that there is always a real risk of having extracapsular disease extension, which is more effectively treated by integrating seed implants with IMRT (or 3D-CRT). Many patients now understand that with IMRT (and especially 4D IG-IMRT with DART) they are afforded the added security of covering possible extracapsular extension while experiencing little to no additional side effects.

What are the Possible Side Effects of Seed Implantation?

Seed implantation involves significantly less risk of long-term complications compared with surgery or conventional EBRT. Side effects with implants are usually mild and reversible. The most common organ system involved with temporary side effects from seed implants is the urinary tract, and this is because the prostate is nestled beneath the bladder and has the urethra running through it. Following implantation, most patients experience increased urinary frequency and urgency, a weakened stream, and occasionally, urinary burning. Fortunately, these symptoms are temporary and resolve as the radioactivity of the seeds dissipates over time.

With palladium implants, the 17-day half-life typically causes about two and a half to four months of some type of urinary symptomology. With the 60-day half-life of iodine implants, urinary symptoms may persist for ten to twelve months. During this period, we do our best to micromanage these urinary symptoms with a variety of medications. The symptoms are in no way debilitating, but rather more of a nuisance, and patients are encouraged to continue their normal level of activity.

While side effects with implantation are usually temporary, there is some risk of more serious, permanent complications, including urinary incontinence (in less than 1% of patients) and erectile dysfunction. When they do occur, such side effects usually appear 6 to 24 months after treatment. As mentioned, patients who have previously undergone TURPs are at higher risk for developing incontinence. Incontinence is a very rare complication associated with implantation therapy in general for patients without TURPs—less than 1% in virtually all studies. But patients with prior TURPs are more likely to develop urinary incontinence, up to 50% according to some researchers. However, brachytherapists who modify their implants and make adjustments for patients with TURPs have reported incontinence in less than 3% of patients (see below, "How are implants modified for patients with prior TURPs?").

Another potential side effect with seeds is irritation to the rectum, although this is uncommon. In my experience with the procedure, I don't have one patient who has had to have a colostomy or who has a persistent rectal ulceration; nor do I have any patients who required urinary diversion because of damage to the urethra. It appears that while the urethra tends to play an important role with seeding in terms of the side effect profile, it generally is able to withstand the dose, and once the seeds decay, the side effects disappear.

What is the Risk of Erectile Dysfunction after Seed Implantation?

Generally speaking, patients having prostate brachytherapy will have erectile dysfunction in about 15% to 20% of cases, although some institutions are reporting higher rates of incidence. Brachytherapy does not appear to produce the steady decline of potency that we have seen with full course external beam radiation through the years. Rather, I have noted not only a leveling off of the potency rate over time after implantation, but even a gradual improvement over time. Essentially, where you are at two to three years after treatment is where you will likely be as far as erectile function, taking into account that patients are getting older and may be taking hypertensive medications, diabetic medications or have other medical problems which could interfere with erectile function over time. Smoking and obesity are also significant causal factors for erectile dysfunction. It should be noted that a diminished ejaculate with a clearer consistency, which may occur after seed implantation, should not be confused with having serious erectile dysfunction, which is the loss of ability to produce and/or sustain an erection sufficient for intercourse.

For those men who lose potency, Viagra® (sildenafil), intracavernosal paparavine, and Prostaglandin E1 injections are very effective. Viagra® has altered the clinical situation considerably. According to one study, for men who are potent at the time of treatment, 92% of patients having seed implants (with or without supplemental external radiation) will maintain erectile function potency. Two additional oral erectile aids, Levitra® (Vardenafil) and Cialis® (Tadalafil) are also available.

It should also be noted that the risk of erectile dysfunction may be reduced with Palladium-103 because of one of its unique physical properties. The radial dose fall-off, that is, the amount of radiation actually delivered at any distance from the Pd-103 seed, is less with palladium than with any other isotope. Therefore, palladium is less likely to over-radiate the neurovascular bundles or proximal penile tissues, both of which affect the ability to have and maintain an erection. Moreover, the dose to the penile bulb approaches nil using 4D IG-IMRT with DART (compared with 40 to 50% with standard IMRT).

How do Seed Implants Affect Sexual Activity?

There are no formal restrictions on sexual activity after seed implantation. A patient can resume sexual activities immediately. Some men may not wish to engage in sex right away as the area may be somewhat irritated. As a safety precaution, patients receiving Pd-103 seeds are advised to utilize a condom for a two to three week period after implantation, so as to avoid the unlikely possibility of ejaculating a seed into his partner. That precaution is extended for patients receiving I-125 seeds because of their longer half-life.

For the majority of patients who retain potency, the major change that we see after implantation is the diminution in the volume of the ejaculate. Shortly after the implant, there may also be a discoloring or a different consistency to the ejaculate. Typically it's described as being clearer and thinner, but most patients have little problem with that as long as they're able to maintain an erection and achieve orgasm.

A patient can have normal sperm after implantation. The testicles are a separate organ from the prostate *per se,* and while there may be a short period of oligospermia (a decrease in the sperm count), a patient very well may have a return of sperm. Although there is little chance that radiation will affect the sperm, attempts to impregnate should be avoided for at least 6 months. Because of the diminished ejaculate, and the change in milieu that the sperm will encounter, the chance of successful impregnation is probably greatly reduced, though several of my patients have success-fully conceived. We counsel our patients that they need to be careful and should not consider themselves to be sterile because of the procedure. At the same time, men wanting to father children should always consider banking sperm before implantation.

What Precautions Should Patients Exercise after the Implant Procedure?

After implantation, patients are advised for the first month not to hold children less than two years of age for extended periods—for hours in a day or for consecutive days. This applies only to Palladium-103 implants, because that isotope has a short half-life and delivers its dose relatively quickly. With Iodine-125 implants, a longer period of restraint needs to be exercised. These restrictions do not mean having no contact. Even during the period immediately after the implant, a patient can have casual contact with children less than two years old. It's perfectly safe for a seeding patient to hold a child his lap for brief periods.

How are Implants Modified for Patients with Prior TURPs?

If a patient has had a TURP, the implant procedure has to be mapped out very carefully and the seeds need to be distributed differently in that particular patient. They have to be positioned in a way that avoids the TURP itself; otherwise, they may be deposited into an empty prostatic cavity and eventually be urinated out. Misplaced seeds may cause potential damage in that way. With these patients, I use a seed loading pattern that is very peripheral to the gland, placing seeds in extracapsular positions and especially avoiding the remaining external sphincter.

The reason that incontinence risks may be higher in these patients is because a TURP typically removes the superior internal sphincter, leaving the patient with only the lower sphincter. The high doses of implant radiation may impair that sphincter's ability to work normally. Another factor to consider is how large the TURP is compared to the size of the prostate. There must be enough prostate tissue around the TURP to anchor the seeds; if the TURP is excessive, there may not be enough tissue for the seeds to adhere. That might be a contraindication to seed implantation, though it's rare that a prior TURP would prevent a patient from being seeded.

What are the Advantages of Palladium-103 over Iodine-125?

The choice of palladium versus iodine is typically based on physician preference, although it is sometimes decided by the patient. While there is some controversy regarding which is the superior source, palladium has long been my isotope of choice, a preference dating back to my experience in the mid-1980s with both Pd-103 and I-125 at New York University Medical Center and Memorial Sloan-Kettering. My research and clinical practice in Tampa during the following decade and my more recent experience in Sarasota have confirmed the advantages of Pd-103 in a large brachytherapy practice.

Radiobiological considerations suggest that palladium would be more effective against rapidly growing, more aggressive cancers (those with higher Gleason scores) as well as low-grade prostate malignancies. While there have been no definitive (prospective, randomized) human clinical trials to date comparing tumor-control rates with Pd-103 and I-125, studies have reported a lower complication rate for Pd-103, as well as a more precipitous fall in PSA levels and reduced incidence of benign PSA "bounce" (see below, What is PSA Bounce?).

Why Should Seed Implants be Done *after* External Radiation?

When external radiation is combined with brachytherapy, the sequence is typically EBRT (preferably IMRT) followed by an implant boost, with the doses of each modality moderated to achieve optimal coverage while at the same time limiting rectal, bladder and urethral doses. The history of the combined approach suggests there may be considerable reason for concern that reversing the sequence (implant first followed by external radiation) may increase the risk of rectal complications, in part because there is a significant interval when patients are receiving simultaneous implant and external radiation.

We have learned that by targeting the tumor and its extensions first with IMRT, with or without hormonal therapy, the seeding procedure is more effective and serves as a boost, while not leaving the migrating cells in the regions outside of the prostate untreated. The surrounding pelvic field is essentially sterilized and cancers are rendered nonviable when IMRT is used before the seed implantation. Some doctors who have treated in the reverse order, implanting seeds before administering external radiation, have reported higher rates of rectal injury. There is also concern that implanting seeds first in intermediate or high grade cancers may spread cancer into the bloodstream. This potential threat is eliminated with the implant-boost approach, because the external radiation has sterilized the peripheral field as well as cancerous cells within the gland prior to the insertion of implant needles.

As noted, traditionally, patients at the Dattoli Cancer Center are treated to an initial dose level of approximately 4500 cGy prior to interstitial brachytherapy. This dose level typically covers not only the prostate, but also potentially surrounding target tissues (including, but not limited to, seminal vesicles, periprostatic lymph nodes, obturator lymph nodes, internal iliac lymph nodes, and even common iliac and para-aortic nodes per individual case as indicated). A 4100 cGy dose was initially chosen since early physics and radiobiologic evaluations performed by physicists at Memorial Sloan-Kettering Cancer Center (MSKCC), especially Dr. Lowell Anderson, suggested that this dose given along with an attenuated dose of palladium-103 of 8000-9000 cGy would not exceed rectal, urethral or bladder tolerances. The 4100 cGy dose has since been increased to 4500 cGy using sophisticated IMRT technologies.

Bear in mind that in the latter 1980s, no one knew the correct doses when combining EBRT and Pd-103. At that time, the Pd-103 isotope was relatively new and Dr. Anderson was instrumental in characterizing the physical parameters and laid the groundwork for clinical models. During that period, I worked closely with Dr. Anderson and other physicists at MSKCC and adopted these dose parameters, and since then I have never had an incidence of rectal fistula or urethral-rectal fistula. The dose of 4500 cGy, however, is insufficient in most cases to eradicate microscopic, and especially potentially macroscopic cancer cells, at a distance from the prostate gland. For this reason, following the implant procedure, the physics/dosimetry staff then generates precise isodose curves emanating from the seed implant (both inside and outside the gland).

The dose projected by the seeds to a given distance from the prostate can then be precisely calculated up to the point of near complete decay of the palladium 103 at the three month mark status post seeding. For this reason, most patients return approximately three months post seeding (at the point of near decay of the isotope) to receive a small number of additional 4D IG-IMRT treatments to peripheral target tissue sites and lymph nodes while blocking the prostate, bladder, rectum, and proximal penile tissues. The individualization of the dose is multifactorial which may include taking into account the size of the gland, stage, size of tumor(s), location of tumor(s), Gleason score, PSA, PAP, prior TURP/TUIP, etc. The optimal dose to target points at distance from the gland, and the subsequent physics analysis will determine the number of treatments necessary to achieve the desired dose. It is to be noted that this methodology has been in place since the mid-1990s, although, is now more liberally utilized with IMRT in view of the safety associated with dose escalation using this newer modality.

What is the Likelihood of Cure with Brachytherapy and IMRT?

The 10-year and 14-year cure rates for brachytherapy or combination therapy using brachytherapy and external radiation (3D-CRT or IMRT) are as good as or better than results achieved with other treatment modalities, including surgical removal of the prostate. Freedom from biochemical failure is typically 90% or higher for low risk patients receiving brachytherapy, while even intermediate and high risk patients may enjoy an approximate 80% freedom from biochemical failure when brachytherapy is combined with external radiation.

The criteria used at my institution for biochemical disease-free survival is quite rigorous. Only patients who achieve and maintain a PSA nadir of 0.2 or less are considered disease-free. After seed implants and external radiation, the prostate is left in place and any remaining normal prostate cells will secrete PSA, so there will be a certain baseline PSA level. I have patients with PSA levels as high as 3.0 that over time have never shown any PSA velocity. Their PSA readings have been stable and not rising for a decade or more; however, when using strict criteria, they are technically not cured, even though most of these patients will probably never have symptoms or die from prostate cancer. As such, the actual cure rate may be somewhat higher than that reported.

What is a PSA Bounce?

About 30% to 40% of patients undergoing seed implantation experience a temporary rise in PSA after an initial decline in their PSA level following treatment. This phenomenon is known as a PSA bounce or flare. It generally occurs approximately 18 to 24 months after treatment and is not caused by a recurrence of cancer, but rather by radiation-induced prostatitis (inflammation of the prostate) with subsequent systemic release of PSA. These patients are still considered disease-free. The rise in PSA may be 0.1 or higher and can sometimes last many months, but it is usually of short duration. Studies have shown that the PSA bounce is more common with younger patients, those who receive higher implant doses, and those with larger prostate glands.

One 40 year old patient saw his PSA rise to 28.6 two years after brachytherapy. This unusually large bounce caused him considerable distress and uncertainty. Repeat staging studies were negative, although urologists wanted to remove his prostate gland. The patient, fortunately, did not have his gland removed and his PSA steadily declined. His most recent PSA reading at ten years is 0.001.

How do Brachytherapy and IMRT Compare with Surgery?

As discussed earlier, treatments can be compared in terms of cure rates and complication rates by evaluating the results obtained at premier medical centers for each treatment specialty. For low risk patients, brachytherapy with or without supplemental IMRT (or 3D-CRT) appears to be comparable to surgery as far as likelihood of cure, but with less risk of serious, long-term complications. For intermediate and high risk patients, a number of recent studies have shown brachytherapy and supplemental IMRT (or 3D-CRT) to be significantly more effective at curing prostate cancer than surgery (Figures 12-13).

One recent study evaluated the peer-reviewed medical literature and concluded that brachytherapy (with or without supplemental EBRT and with or without hormonal therapy) was superior to radical surgery for the treatment of high risk patients. The abstract reads as follows: "High-risk prostate cancer represents a therapeutic challenge for both the urologist and radiation oncologist. Biochemical outcomes with radical prostatectomy and external-beam radiation therapy are poor in this subset of patients. These unfavorable results have led some to believe that high-risk prostate cancer is not curable with conventional treatment approaches, which has been an impetus for many of the current trials using neoadjuvant chemotherapy and prostatectomy. With the established efficacy of interstitial brachytherapy, these efforts are likely excessive. Most modern trials indicate excellent biochemical control rates among

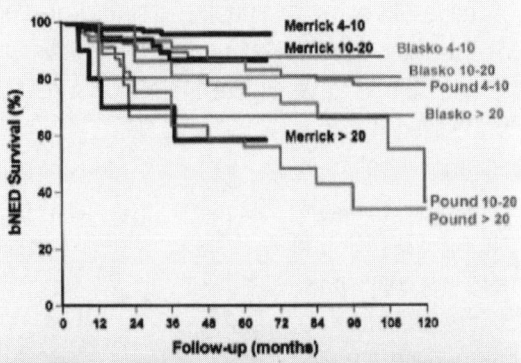

Figure 12–Permanent Prostate Brachytherapy compared to Prostatectomy. Biochemical disease free survival (bNED) for selected prostatectomy (Pound et al) and brachytherapy series (Blasko et al, Merrick et al) stratified by pretreatment prostate specific antigen level (J of Brachy Int., Vol. 17, July-Sept. 2001, 193).

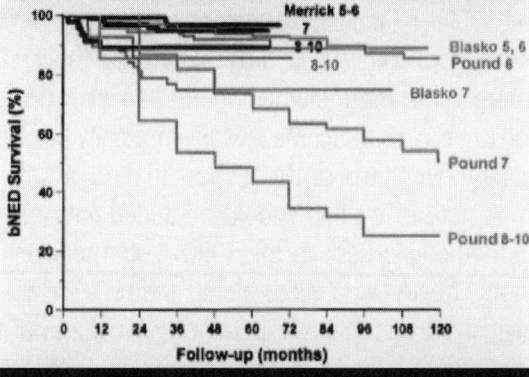

Figure 13–Permanent Prostate Brachytherapy compared to Prostatectomy. Biochemical disease-free (bNED) survival for selected prostatectomy (Pound et al) and brachytherapy series (Blasko et al, Merrick et al) stratified by Gleason score of at least 5 (J of Brachy Int., Vol. 17, July-Sept. 2001, 193).

high-risk patients treated with an aggressive locoregional approach that includes brachytherapy. A thoughtful review of the literature would suggest that interstitial brachytherapy offers a therapeutic advantage over other local treatment modalities and should be considered standard treatment for aggressive organ-confined prostate cancer" (Bittner N, et al, "Interstitial brachytherapy should be standard of care for treatment of high-risk prostate cancer," Oncology, Williston Park, 2008 Aug;22 (9):995-1004).

The results of my own published studies are consistent with those reported by the brachytherapy teams described above, showing a similar plateau in the disease-free curve (Figure 14). My personal series dates from 1991 with Pd-103 seed implantation and supplemental external radiation, utilizing 3D-CRT and more recently IMRT for the treatment of intermediate and high risk patients. The overall actuarial freedom from biochemical failure at 10 years was 79% in patients

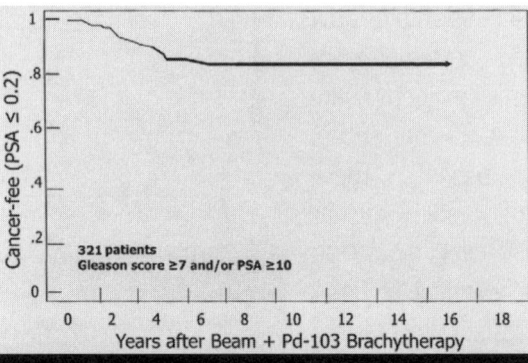

Figure 14—Freedom from biochemical progression for 321 patients with PSA ≥10 and/or Gleason score ≥7 treated with external radiation followed by Pd-103 brachytherapy.

having locally advanced, high risk prostate cancer. That number has actually improved to more than 82% with patients who have now been followed for 16 years or more. Meanwhile, morbidity has been limited to temporary urinary symptoms, similar to those that occur with seed implants alone.

A note of caution should be added with regard to seed implants as monotherapy. Back in the 1990s, intermediate risk patients were commonly treated with seeds alone, and now we are seeing a small percentage of these patients experiencing biochemical failure beyond 8 years. This would indicate that the combined approach of seed implants with supplemental external radiation is a more effective protocol for patients at the intermediate risk level.

Our success with higher risk patients is indicative of an important area where brachytherapy and 4D IG-IMRT offer significant advantages over surgery. From a surgical perspective, it's very difficult if not impossible to cure stage T3 malignancies, and it's very difficult to cure patients having Gleason scores in the 8 to 10 range and even PSAs greater than 20. But we have had a very successful run using external radiation for about four to five weeks, and then adding the implant boost using Pd-103 brachytherapy about four weeks later. This integrated approach (with or without brief hormonal therapy) has been able to cure some cancers which were formerly deemed to be incurable with surgery or any other treatment option.

As mentioned, even patients who have evidence of lymph node involvement are now being treated. This group of patients is also treated with hormonal agents. Combined hormone blockade is followed by 4D IG-IMRT to target not only the prostate but also the periprostatic tissues and the lymph node bearing sites. Then finally the seeds are implanted where most of the tumor volume is, namely in the prostate itself. Having treated patients with lymph node cancer successfully, we are moving up the ladder in terms of the stage of the disease that can be conquered.

What is Proton Beam Radiation Therapy and how does it Compare to Other Forms of Radiation?

Radiation therapy in all its forms utilizes atomic or subatomic particles: electrons, protons, neutrons and photons, which include x-rays and gamma rays. These particles differ in terms of charge, mass and other physical characteristics. Like visible light, the energy of conventional x-ray radiation takes the form of photons. Radiation therapies utilizing proton and neutron beams have been developed in the hope that they might offer some advantage over conventional photon beams. Protons and neutrons are generated by proton accelerators rather than the linear accelerators that are used to generate photons.

Each type of radiation therapy delivers a dose of highly energized particles that interact in various ways with the tissue they traverse. In the case of x-rays and protons, a process called ionization causes electrons to be displaced in the atoms of DNA molecules in cancer cells. This interaction damages the DNA and causes cell death. The strategy of targeting tumors with cancer-killing doses of radiation is essentially the same regardless of which kind of radiation is used.

Unlike other forms of radiation like x-rays that begin releasing their energy as soon as they enter the body, protons travel through bodily tissues initially releasing very little energy, but at a certain calculable point, the energy that the beam delivers rises dramatically to a peak, known as the Bragg peak. The Bragg peak is like the focus of a magnifying lens, and allows the radiation to be targeted to the site of the tumor. Protons may appear at first to have some theoretical advantage over photons because they can be accurately focused to release most of their ionizing energy at a certain depth to encompass a calculated tumor volume, while avoiding nearby healthy organs. By contrast, the depth at which photons deposit their maximal energy is determined by the energy levels of the photons and can range from the skin surface to a depth of approximately 5 centimeters.

The radiobiological effect (RBE) of protons in high doses is nearly identical to the RBE of high-energy photons utilized with IMRT. However, with its highly sophisticated beam arrangements and state-of-the-art prostate immobilization, IMRT allows for the delivery of higher doses than protons. Several published studies have already demonstrated the advantages of IMRT over 3D-CRT at high dose levels, and proton therapy at this time does not deliver higher doses than 3D-CRT. The preponderance of data suggests that higher doses lead to higher cure rates, regardless of the type of radiation utilized. It appears unlikely that researchers using protons will be able to safely escalate doses as high as those now achieved with IMRT, or the even higher doses delivered when IMRT is combined with a seed implant boost.

Proton beam radiation therapy (PBRT) is available at only a limited number of institutions in the U.S. PBRT is usually performed on an outpatient basis over a period of 7 to 8 weeks (35 to 40 sessions). Protons are sometimes combined with a reduced course of conventional radiation. Proton therapy is FDA and Medicare approved, but with a cost as high as $160,00, roughly four to five times that of the most sophisticated photon therapy (4D IG-IMRT with DART).

Proton therapy causes significantly fewer complications than traditional external radiation therapy, though its precision in sparing healthy tissues is surpassed by IMRT and/or brachytherapy using the most advanced technologies and in the most skilled hands. About half of all proton therapy patients experience some urinary discomfort two to three weeks into treatment. Those symptoms usually dissipate 2 to 3 three weeks after completing therapy. About 20% of patients develop intermittent rectal bleeding, which may occur 9 to 12 months after treatment and persist episodically for a year or two. A proton therapy patient has between a 30% and 50% chance of experiencing problems with potency, roughly equivalent to the results obtained with nerve-sparing prostatectomies. When erectile dysfunction occurs after proton therapy, it usually happens 9 to 12 months after treatment.

The June 2008 issue of *Oncology Journal* (Vol, 33, No. 7, pp. 748-753) presents the most recent assessment of the heated contentions between proponents of protons and photons. The article is authored by radiation oncologists at Harvard Medical School (Nguyen PL, et al) the first institution in the world to utilize proton therapy (primarily for small brain tumors). The abstract follows: "There is a growing interest in the use of proton therapy for the treatment of many cancers. While much evidence supports this notion in context of many oncologic sites, only limited clinical data have compared protons to photon in prostate cancer. Therefore, the increasing enthusiasm for the use of protons in prostate cancer has aroused considerable concern. Some have questioned its ability to limit morbidity. Theoretical concerns over potential additional risks for developing secondary malignancies (ie, cancer in other areas of the body), as well as promoting hip fractures. In this article, we review the current status of the evidence supporting the use of protons in prostate cancer and discuss the active controversies that surround this modality."

The study concludes, "While there is growing enthusiasm for the use of protons in the treatment of prostate cancer, a review of the literature suggests there is so far no clear evidence to show that proton therapy would be superior to highly conformal photon treatments [such as IMRT]."

Based on the literature, we believe that the best use for protons is in the treatment of tiny brain tumors, and not for treating a gland the size of the prostate. Because protons travel in tiny, straight beams, they must be "scattered" to form a large enough beam to treat the entire area of the prostate. With what is referred to as "passive scattering," or "passive modulation" (the most common proton delivery method utilized), "scattering foils" are added to produce a beam of large enough size to cover the entire target. Unfortunately, once the proton beam encounters the filter or scanner, it becomes cone-shaped and results in spreading the radiation dose outside the target area. In other words, the beam cannot be manipulated into a spherical shape as can be done with the photon beam (or IMRT) using multi-leaf collimators.

Eric J. Hall, D.Phil, D.Sc, of Columbia University, widely regarded as the world's premiere radiobiologist, writing in The International Journal of Radiation Oncology, Biology and Physics (2006;65:1-7), states: "Protons emerging from a cyclotron form a narrow pencil beam. To cover a treatment field of practical size, the beam must be either scattered by a foil or scanned. Passive scanning is by far the simplest technique but suffers the disadvantage of increased total-body effective dose to the patient… Passive modulation results in [neutron] doses distant from the field edge that are 10 times higher than those characteristic of IMRT." Dr. Hall also observes, "…the scattering foil becomes a source of neutrons, which results in a total-body dose to the patient."

Because of this widening cone-shaped bean, the side effects with protons will be greater even at lower dose levels than with our high energy photons, the exact opposite of what many patients are currently told. It should be noted that protons are unable to target specific tumor sites within the prostate gland to higher dose levels, while lacking the ability to minimize doses to the urethra. Protons also cannot be utilized to target lymph nodes. In proton therapy there is always a need for a "compensating filter" in order to expand the beam width to treat the prostate to appropriate dose levels. In doing so, control over the modulation of the beam is lost and it becomes impossible to target small areas within the prostate to receive lower or higher doses as is possible with 4D IG-IMRT (that is, dose escalation or dose demodulation). Therefore, with protons, the entire prostate receives the same doses and this dose is minimal compared to what can be achieved with 4D IG-IMRT. While the overall dose to the prostate may look the same as with proton therapy, the ability to control the dose to the critical structures within the target (prostate) is lost.

These functional results from proton filtering or scanning make 4D IG-IMRT a more versatile and therefore arguably superior treatment to proton therapy. In addition, because of the need for the "compensating filter," the normal adjacent tissues, including the bladder and rectum through which the proton beam enters the pelvis, receive a far higher dose than with 4D IG-IMRT. The latter modality allows for "inverse treatment planning," which is utilized for the initial IMRT planning phase. Inverse treatment planning provides the oncologist with the ability to plan for and control the amount of radiation received by the tissues surrounding the prostate while maximizing the dose to the prostate.

Thereafter, a number of technological advances mentioned previously, including but not limited to SonArray, Cone Beam Tomography, Exact Couch™, Portal Vision, On-Board Imaging, and Respiratory Gating, are combined to allow for the analysis of organ motion in real-time (the 4th dimension) to achieve unsurpassed accuracy. As described earlier, once the motion is detected, numerous software programs activate to adapt the radiation to target the organ site which may have moved. This is true Dynamic Adaptive Radiotherapy (DART). Using gating technologies, 4D IG-IMRT can even hit a continually moving target! This ability to optimize and adapt to changes is the basis for DART, and none of this is even remotely possible with protons.

What is Neutron Beam Therapy and how does it Compare with Other Forms of Radiation?

The basic effect of ionizing radiation is to disrupt the ability of cells to divide and grow by damaging their DNA strands. With photons and protons, the damage is done primarily by activated radical ions produced by atomic interactions involving electrons orbiting the nucleus of the atom. Because of the nature of these characteristic interactions, photon and proton radiation are referred to as low linear energy transfer (low LET) radiation. With neutron radiation, the damage to the DNA is done primarily by nuclear interactions. Neutrons are referred to as high linear energy transfer (high LET) radiation. Tumor cells damaged by high LET radiation (neutrons) are less able to repair themselves and continue to grow than are tumor cells damaged by low LET radiation (photons and protons).

In addition, unlike low LET photons and protons, neutrons do not depend on oxygen to damage the DNA in cancer cells and cause cell death. Therefore, neutron beam therapy may have a certain theoretical advantage over conventional photon radiation because high LET neutrons may be more effective against large, bulky tumors that typically have low oxygen levels (hypoxic) near the center of their mass. This characteristic of neutrons might afford some benefit when treating these larger tumors that are more resistant to low LET radiation and to hormonal therapy.

The radiobiological effect of neutrons is so high that the required prescription dose is about one-third the dose required with photons or protons. As such, a full course of neutron therapy is carried out with only 10 to 12 treatments, compared to 30 to 40 treatments needed for conventional x-ray radiation. Neutrons are sometimes combined with a reduced course of standard radiation therapy. Clinical trials of neutrons have suggested that they may be more effective against advanced prostate cancers than is conventional radiation; however, these results are still considered short-term. It should also be noted that because neutrons are such a highly penetrating form of radiation, they have also been demonstrated to result in a far greater risk of complications than conventional radiation therapy.

What are the Treatment Options if External Radiation Fails?

Patients who are not cured by any of the various forms of external radiation therapy have several options for salvage therapy, including radical surgery. As mentioned, the operation to remove the prostate is more difficult after radiation. Many doctors do not recommend salvage prostatectomy because of their own limited experience. They will inform the patient that the risk of complications is high, while the likelihood of cure is relatively low. Nonetheless, this remains a viable option in experienced surgical hands.

A second treatment with radiation is usually not advised since the first course of radiation did not cure the cancer and the risk of complications is high. There has been, however, a growing interest in treating failed external radiation patients with brachytherapy, since seed implant radiation can be focused on the prostate, with less risk of damage to the rectum and surrounding tissue. One recent study reported that as many as 50% of these salvage brachytherapy patients were disease-free at 5 years.

Cryosurgery is a primary treatment method that involves the insertion of freezing probes into the prostate to kill cancerous tissue. This technique has also been used as a salvage therapy for locally recurrent prostate cancer after failed radiation, though there is little published data available. One study reported a disease-free survival rate of 74% after two years, but with a high rate of complications such as incontinence and erectile dysfunction. This incontinence rate is dramatically reduced in experienced hands.

If a man's PSA after external radiation (or brachytherapy) rises only very slowly over a period of one to three years, then the cancer may still be confined within the prostate. These patients have the most options of patients who fail with radiation, including watchful waiting. A number of studies have shown that there are patients with biopsy-detected local recurrence who have survived 10 years or more without experiencing any progression of the disease. However, more aggressive tumors with Gleason scores of 7 to 10 may secrete little PSA, and even a slow PSA rise may be significant with respect to tumor growth and cancer spread.

In addition to salvage treatments like brachytherapy, surgery and cryosurgery, there are also the options of hormonal therapy or orchiectomy (surgical castration). The same considerations that apply to hormonal therapy after failed surgery apply to hormonal therapy for men with local or distant cancer recurrence after radiation. Some studies suggest that men treated with a combination of hormones and radiation as their initial treatment have a reduced rate of failure. However, initial radical prostatectomy coupled with hormones have not demonstrated a similar benefit.

With the object of shutting down the body's production of testosterone completely, many doctors combine drugs like Lupron® (or Eligard® or Zoladex® or TRELSTAR®) with Casodex® (or Eulexin®), which together provide a total blockage against the male hormones that nourish prostate cancer. For many men, the use of this type of combination hormonal therapy to achieve a castration level of testosterone that may slow the progression of the disease is preferable to undergoing surgical castration (orchiectomy), which is a less expensive way to achieve the same end. In addition, unlike surgical castration, this form of medical castration is reversible and may be used intermittently. The patients may be on hormones 6 to 12 months, and then completely off hormones until the PSA reaches a predetermined value. This allows for recovery of the male bodily functions.

What are the Treatment Options if Brachytherapy Fails?

Patients who have had seed implantation without initial success have the option of being re-seeded. Although long term results are not yet available, this approach appears to be promising, and typically involves using a different isotope the second time around. If the patient was first implanted with iodine, then palladium might be used as a salvage therapy in the hope that the cancer will be more sensitive to the second isotope. If the first implant was technically mishandled, then a second implant affords the opportunity of correcting misplacements that may have caused underdosing. In some cases, HDR temporary implants may be used if permanent implants fail.

Brachytherapy patients who experience treatment failure also have the salvage options of surgery, cryosurgery, hormonal therapy, and watchful waiting. In some cases, several months of hormonal therapy may be prescribed to reduce the size of the tumor prior to salvage therapy with either surgery or cryosurgery. Patients may also consider biothermy, which combines cryosurgery and hyperthermia. Focal cryosurgery may also be a viable salvage option, especially if the recurrent cancer is confined to one lobe of the gland. High Intensity Frequency Ultrasound is another option, and as noted, researchers are working on vaccines for which there are clinical trials underway.

A Summary of the 16-year Data

The following summary is based on a Dattoli series that was presented at a recent ASCO meeting (February, 2009). The summary also draws on another published series, *Long-term Prostate Cancer Control using Palladium-103 Brachytherapy and External Beam Radiotherapy in Patients with a High Likelihood of Extracapsular Cancer Extension* by Michael Dattoli, MD, Richard Sorace, MD, Jennifer Cash, ARNP and Kent Wallner, MD (*Urology*, 2007 Feb; 69(2):334-7).

The bottom line in both studies is these are patients who were at high risk, with a high likelihood of extra-capsular extension. These patients were treated with 3D-Conformal Radiation followed by seed implantation, with large margins. The study was by a single author doing the implants, but the biochemical data was independently reviewed by the University of Washington, and all the slides were re-reviewed by the University of Washington, which adds an element of security to the data. Clinical stage was not included because the doctors at the University of Washington couldn't do a digital rectal exam on these patients due to distance.

The 16-year Data–*Summary*

Materials and Methods
321 Consecutive Patients treated by one author (M.D.)—157 intermediate risk and 164 high risk.

Selection Criteria
NCCN Guidelines

Radiation Treatment Regimen
➤ 3D-CRT Dose: 4140cGy Media n (Range 39 Gy–54 Gy)

➤ Pd-103 Dose: 8000-9000 Minimum Peripheral Dose (pre-NIST-99)

➤ Source Strength: 1.4 mCi Median (Range 1.1-1.6 mCi)

➤ Clinical Pd-103 Target Volume: extended 0.5 – 1.0 cm, anterolaterally to the TRUS prostate margin

➤ Patients were followed at 3, 6 and 12 months, and every 6-12 months thereafter

➤ Definition of biochemical success: PSA ≤ 0.2 ng/ml, nadir +2 and ASTRO Consensus Definition

➤ Follow-up saturation prostate biopsies were performed on all failing patients

➤ Biochemical data independently re-reviewed and analyzed by Kent Wallner, MD (Univ. of Washington)

➤ Original biopsy slides re-reviewed by Lawrence True, MD (Univ. of Washington)

➤ Clinical stage was not included in final data analysis to reduce subjectivity

Patient Characteristics
➤ Mean PSA 19.4 (1.6–147)

➤ Median PSA 16.4

➤ 218 Patients had Gleason Score 7-10

➤ 203 Patients had PSA > 10

➤ 79 Patients had elevated PAPs

> 141 Patients had Clinical Stage T2C

> 127 Patients had Clinical Stage T3

Follow-up

> 16 year actuarial, Median 10.3 years

> 143 Patients received a median of 4 months neo-adjuvant or adjuvant therapy

Results

> PAP was the strongest predictor of failure (p= 0.0001), followed by Gleason Score (p< 0.001) and PSA (p=0.03)

> Hormones conferred no survival advantage (p=0.4) although patients receiving hormones had the most adverse features

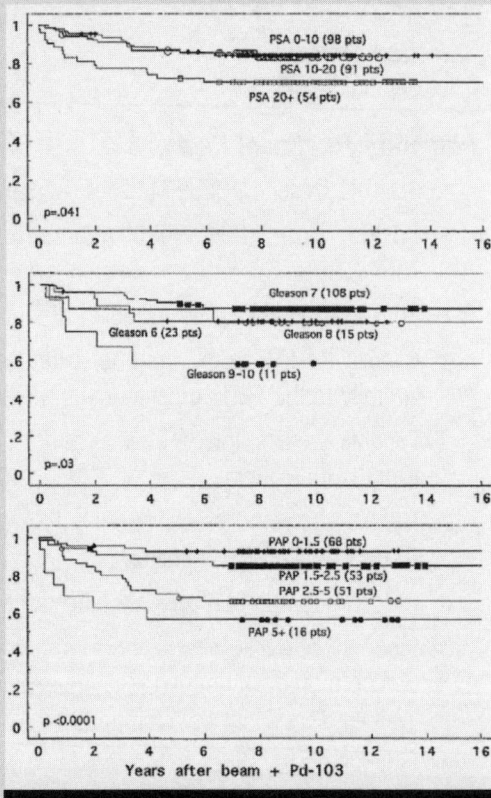

These three graphs show the freedom of biographical progression of the disease out to 16 years stratified by PSA, Gleason Score, and PAP.

> 82% overall actuarial freedom from biochemical progress at 16 years using strict PSA nadir of ≤0.2 ng/ml (Freedom from failure calculated by method of Kaplan-Meier. Difference between groups were determined by the log rank or students' t-test) (86% cancer specific survival; 89% intermediate and 74% high risk)

> The absolute risk of failure fell to 1% beyond 5 years after treatment

➤ Treatment morbidity was limited to RTOG grade 1-2 symptoms. No patients experienced grade 3-4 toxicity. (One patient who had both a TURP and TUIP developed low-volume stress incontinence.) No patient developed rectal ulceration

➤ All failing patients underwent prostatic biopsies. There were no pathologically documented local failures

Conclusions

➤ Patients having high risk prostate cancer may enjoy long-term bio-chemical freedom even when using strict PSA nadirs

➤ Morbidity has been very acceptable

➤ Despite the aggressive nature of this study group, no local failures have been documented

➤ It is encouraging that the failure rate decreased to near zero with follow-up beyond 5 years

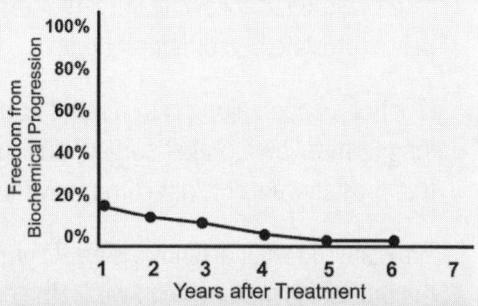

This graph shows the likelihood of subsequent bio-chemical failure versus years after treatment. These results are encouraging because as time goes on fewer and fewer patients experience biochemical failure, indicated by a PSA greater than 0.2.

➤ These results appear superior to surgery, aggressive external beam radiotherapy (including full course IMRT ± hormones, protons/ neutrons or combined radiation methods using other isotopes ± hormones) in this high risk group

➤ We attribute these exceedingly favorable results, in part, to our effort to achieve wide brachytherapy treatment margins. This is accomplished by using highly peripheral and extra-capsular source placement

➤ PD-103 appears to be the isotope best suited for high-risk cancers

Independent Review and Summary of 14-year Data

Charles E. Myers Jr., M.D., founder and director of the American Institute for Diseases of the Prostate, recently reviewed our 14 year series following high risk patients (*Prostate Forum*, Vol. 10, No. 6, March 2008). Dr. Myers highlighted the following points of that study:

"Many men with intermediate to high-risk prostate cancer treated with radiation to the prostate gland and pelvic lymph nodes with external beam radiation and seeds remain free of disease out to 14 years.

"Men who recur following surgery most commonly recur in the pelvis (prostate bed or lymph nodes).

"Dattoli's paper, along with a number of other papers reporting long term follow up after surgery and radiation, clearly indicates that prostate cancer is not commonly metastatic at diagnosis.

"Prostate cancer at diagnosis is most commonly either localized to the prostate gland or spread within the pelvis and thus potentially accessible to radiation or surgery.

"Radiation therapy is consistently more effective when combined with androgen withdrawal. Faced with these facts, I can only conclude that radiation therapy can kill prostate cancer stem cells or in some way arrest their ability to go on to establish metastatic disease."

Dr. Myers also summarized the results as follows: "Dr. Dattoli's paper reports on the effectiveness of 3D conformal radiation therapy plus palladium seed implantation in a group of men with intermediate or high-risk disease. There are several important aspects to Dattoli's paper, but the most important is that it represents a follow-up extending out to 14 years after treatment. After the sixth year, Dattoli's team saw very few relapses, so the number of patients disease-free at 14 years very likely represents an accurate estimate of the proportion of patients cured. Their results are quite remarkable when you consider the seriousness of the cancer treated."

CHAPTER SEVEN

CRYOSURGERY, HYPERTHERMIA AND HIFU THERAPIES

What is Cryosurgery?

Cryosurgery (also called cryotherapy or cryoablation) uses the process of freezing and thawing to destroy cancer cells. The technique has been in use for some time for the treatment of cervical cancer, as well as malignancies of the head, neck, and skin. Early attempts at prostate cryosurgery were associated with an unacceptably high rate of complications, but the advent of transrectal ultrasound has improved cryosurgical results for the treatment of early stage prostate cancer.

Current cryosurgical technique involves subjecting prostate tissue to extremely cold temperatures (-40° or less) with the use of probes containing liquid nitrogen and more recently Argon gas. The cryoprobes are needles inserted through the perineum and into the prostate gland. The probes create ice balls that destroy both cancerous and normal prostate tissue. The urethra is protected by an indwelling catheter through which a warm saline solution is circulated.

Ultrasound, CT scans or MRI may be used to guide the placement of 6 to 8 probes, and to carefully control the amount of tissue frozen. Temperature probes (thermocouples) within and around the gland monitor the freezing process. The procedure may be repeated two to three times to achieve maximum destruction or ablation of the gland. Several months of hormonal therapy may be used to reduce the size of the gland prior to treatment.

Cryosurgery may offer certain advantages over radical surgery. The freezing procedure does not involve any cutting and is performed on an outpatient basis under local or general anesthesia. Unlike surgery, cryosurgery can be repeated, however, this may not be an advantage, as the object of treatment is to eradicate the cancer initially, once and for all. Many patients are circumspect about a therapy that may only be temporary, and recurrent cancers, when they occur, are typically more aggressive.

Prostate tissue destroyed by the cryosurgery procedure is not removed, but is absorbed by the body. Recovery time is brief, and serious complications in recent years have been comparable to surgery and conventional external beam radiation. Because the procedure typically damages or destroys the neurovascular bundles, most cryosurgery patients are rendered impotent by the procedure. Patients who choose cryosurgery should therefore be prepared to deal with erectile dysfunction.

Another source of concern about cryosurgery stems from the fact that studies have shown that as many as 20% to 30% of patients have cancer that involves the urethra or the tissue immediately surrounding the urethra. Because cryosurgery entails warming the urethra, there is some likelihood that cancer in this area will not be destroyed by the procedure. Additionally, patients who have cancers involving the apex (bottom portion) of the prostate are likely to suffer incontinence since the external sphincter is invariably affected.

What Patients are Eligible for Cryosurgery?

The procedure does not involve much physical stress and is well tolerated by most men, although cryosurgery does typically require two to four hours utilizing techniques such as rectal warming (whereby saline is instilled between the rectum and prostate). Candidates for cryosurgery as a primary treatment should be limited to those patients with early stage prostate cancer (T2 or less). Men with more advanced cancer are less likely to be cured because the cryoprobes are only effective at killing cancer within the prostate and at the periphery of the gland. As discussed previously, cryosurgery is also being used as a salvage therapy for patients with locally recurrent cancer after radiation and has shown promising results (Bahn et al, "Salvage cryosurgery for recurrent prostate cancer after radiation therapy: a seven-year follow-up," Clin Prosate Cancer, 2003 Sep;2(2):111-4).

What are the Risks of Complications after Cryosurgery?

As mentioned, most cryosurgery patients experience erectile dysfunction. According to the published reports, the likelihood of other complications varies considerably and probably reflects the skills and experience of the cryosurgeons and differences in the equipment used. The freezing process may damage the bladder and intestines, leading to pain, a burning sensation, and the need to empty the bladder and bowels often. In addition, a fistula (an abnormal opening or passage) between the rectum and bladder develops in about 2% of men after cryosurgery even in experienced hands. This problem may require surgical repair.

Approximately 50% of patients experience swelling of the penis and scrotum after cryosurgery, usually lasting a couple of weeks. Most men recover normal bowel and bladder function. Approximately 10% to 15% of patients experience sloughing of dead tissue into the urethra. When this occurs, a TURP is usually performed to remove the excess tissue in order to prevent urethral blockage. The TURP may increase incontinence rates considerably.

What is the Likelihood of Cure with Cryosurgery?

Early results with cryosurgery have been mixed. There is no long-term data to suggest that cryosurgery is superior to either radiation therapy or surgery. One 5-year multi-institutional study reported no progression of the disease in 45%, 71% and 76% of high, intermediate and low-risk patients respectively—an overall success rate of 63% (Long JP, Bahn D, Lee F, et al, Urology 57:518-523, 2001).

More recently, Dr. Duke Bahn reported results on a relatively new approach with cryosurgery, known as "focal prostate cryoablation" (Bahn DK, et al, J Endourol. 2006 Sep;20(9):688-92). This technique involves partial ablation of the gland with ice and is aimed at treating the primary tumor while sparing healthy tissue in the gland and surrounding structures. Some cryosurgeons refer to this technique as "prostate lumpectomy," and patients eligible for this approach are usually limited to those having unilateral prostate cancer (tumor confined to one lobe). One of the goals of limiting the treatment area is to reduce side effects such as erectile dysfunction and incontinence. As mentioned, focal prostate cryoablation has shown some promise as a salvage therapy after failed radiation.

With regard to the focal therapy concept, I have serious reservations about its use as a primary treatment. The problem with prostate cancer tends to be the location where most cancers begin, which is the periphery of the gland. The vast majority of cancers begin there in the peripheral zone, depending on the study you read, 70% to 95%. That's not to say that they can't occur elsewhere, but if they do occur in the central zone for example, it's not such an issue. Those cancers tend to be clinically insignificant. It's the ones that occur at the posterior boundary that present most of the problems. Prostate lumpectomy is an area where I take issue, because if we are talking about prostate cancer, I believe it's a multi-focal disease. Focal cryoblation may have applicability as a salvage therapy where the recurrent cancer is locally confined to one lobe, but as a primary therapy, the focal approach appears to be seriously flawed.

To expand on the analogy to women with breast cancer having a lumpectomy, patients routinely receive external beam radiation therapy following the lumpectomy, because of the multi-centricity of the disease. With prostate cancer, even if there is no cancer found outside the primary tumor by saturation biopsies, all of the cells in the gland have been under the same environment and milieu as the cancerous cells, and they will eventually succumb to the disease. I say this because when we began the modern era twenty years ago, we tried this focal approach with brachytherapy, limiting ourselves to just implanting the nodule. We would implant to this localized area, and lo and behold, the PSA would decline, only to find about a year or year and a half later, the PSA was back up again, and the cancer reoccurred somewhere else in the gland. So I will challenge the notion of lumpectomy to the prostate as a long term solution. I want to emphasize the long term because this is a long term disease.

Cryosurgeons often say that an advantage to their approach is that they can re-treat. This will surely bring them more repeat cases, though patients should be very aware that their best chance of getting rid of the disease altogether is with their initially chosen treatment, and they should never be thinking about the ease of re-treatment as is often touted with cryosurgery. One reason is that recurrences are often far more aggressive (either having been around for some time untreated or only partially treated or having mutated) and are commonly associated with distant spread of the disease.

It is still too early to judge the true effectiveness of conventional cryosurgery or the focal technique as a cure for prostate cancer. Some cryosurgeons point out that results have lagged behind refinements in the procedure, such as the relatively recent use of Argon as a coolant and the use of a template similar to that used for brachytherapy to guide the cryoprobes. Progress has made evaluation of cryosurgery problematic because the equipment and techniques vary substantially at those centers offering the procedure. Patients who are inclined toward this treatment are advised to choose one of the premier cryosurgeons with published results.

What is Hyperthermia and How is it Used in Treating Prostate Cancer?

Interstitial Hyperthermia is a therapeutic approach that utilizes heat to kill cancer cells. The strategy is to apply heat selectively to the prostate gland while cooling surrounding structures. This technique is under investigation in clinical trials primarily with patients who have recurrent or locally advanced prostate cancer. In these cases hyperthermia may be combined with external radiation and/or hormonal therapy and/or chemotherapy.

A variety of technologies have been employed to deliver heat ablation, including microwaves and more recently high energy radio waves (sometimes referred to as radiothermia or radio frequency ablation, RFA).

Interstitial Microwave Hyperthermia has been studied extensively in the treatment of BPH and its safety is well established. One recent application of microwaves for the treatment of prostate cancer utilized magnetic fluid nanoparticles, whereby nanoparticle suspensions were injected transperineally into the prostate under transrectal ultrasound and fluoroscopic guidance. Other approaches utilize microwave radiating 'helical antennae' inserted percutaneously (via needle puncture). This procedure also relies on transrectal ultrasound guidance.

The results with hyperthermia have shown promise, especially when combined with other modalities. The cancercidal effects of radiation and certain drugs may be enhanced by increased temperatures. The goal with hyperthermia is to selectively achieve temperatures within the prostate between approximately 40 and 44 degrees Celsius. Studies are also underway on a treatment protocol known as biothermy, which involves combining hyperthermia with cryosurgery. It should be noted that there is an extensive body of literature spanning four decades on using hyperthermia for treating cancer. It has fallen out of favor because cancers rapidly recur after obtaining seemingly complete clinical remission. As with other treatments, patients who pursue hyperthermia and related therapies are advised to find a physician with experience, rather than one who is just starting on the learning curve.

What is High Intensity Focused Ultrasound (HIFU)?

Like hyperthermia, High Intensity Focused Ultrasound (also referred to as High Intensity Frequency Ultrasound, or HIFU) uses heat to kill cancer cells. HIFU utilizes high energy ultrasound generated from a probe inserted in the rectum while the patient is under a spinal or general anesthetic. The endorectal probe incorporates an ultrasound scanner and an HIFU treatment applicator. The sound waves from the applicator are focused on selected sections of the prostate, which heat up, to between 85 and 100 degrees Celsius, destroying tissue in the target area while sparing healthy surrounding tissue. Using a computer screen, doctors guide the ultrasound beam away from nerves essential for erections and for bladder and bowel control. As a result the risk of incontinence and impotence may be minimized.

A 2007 study from the Georgetown University School of Medicine summarized the early results with HIFU as follows: "High-intensity focused ultrasound (HIFU) has emerged in the past decade as a new addition to the armamentarium of treatment options for prostate cancer. Clinical studies have investigated its use as a treatment for clinically localized disease and as salvage therapy in the setting of failure after external beam radiotherapy. Additional studies with long-term follow-up are needed to further evaluate the cancer control and quality of life outcomes of this new therapeutic modality" (Lynch JH, Loeb S, *Curr Oncol* Rep. 2007 May;9(3):222-5).

A more recent study in France has cast serious doubt on the efficacy of HIFU, reporting "overall disappointing results"–demonstrating that a good initial response (seemingly complete remission) is often followed by rapidly recurring cancer, especially in intermediate and high risk patients (Misraï V, et al, "Oncologic control provided by HIFU therapy as single treatment in men with clinically localized prostate cancer," World J Urol. 2008 Jun 26). This study reported that overall 43.7% of patients experienced biochemical recurrence in less than 5 years. Given these results and the lack of of long term studies, HIFU should be reserved as a salvage therapy option for patients who have failed radiation.

CHAPTER EIGHT

TREATING METASTATIC DISEASE

What Treatments are Used When Cancer Spreads Beyond the Prostate?

When cancer spreads beyond the prostate gland, it generally goes to the pelvic lymph nodes first, and then spreads to distant sites in the body such as the bones. Because of the slow progression of prostate cancer, some men can live for many years even after cancer has metastasized to the lymph nodes or bones. As discussed, significant progress has been made using the combined protocol of brachytherapy and IMRT (with or without brief hormonal therapy) for treating high risk patients with locally advanced disease (seminal vesicle or regional lymph node involvement).

Unfortunately, once prostate cancer has spread beyond the lymph nodes to the bones or other distant sites, the disease is not considered curable by any of the primary therapies. However, a recent study by researchers at the University of Rochester reported promising results treating advanced disease with limited metastatic bone lesions (Singh D, et al, "Is there a favorable subset of patients with prostate cancer who develop oligometastases?" Int J Radiat Oncol Biol Phys. 2004 Jan 1;58 (1):3-10). That study concludes, "Patients with < or =5 metastatic sites had significantly better survival rates than patients with >5 lesions. Because existing sites of metastatic disease may be the primary sites of origin for additional metastases, our findings suggest that early detection and aggressive treatment of patients with a small number of metastatic lesions is worth testing as an approach to improving long-term survival."

Patients with metastatic disease are most often treated by hormonal therapy to temporarily halt the progression of the disease and to relieve symptoms. Patients with advanced prostate cancer may also be treated with various investigational drugs and therapies, or they may opt for watchful waiting.

What is Hormonal Therapy and How Does it Work?

Hormonal therapy, or androgen deprivation therapy (ADT), is a standard treatment for those patients whose cancer has spread beyond the prostate gland. At present, nothing works better for advanced prostate cancer than hormonal therapy. If after radiation therapy or surgery or cryosurgery, there is evidence of a rising PSA (biochemical failure) or a positive biopsy, hormonal therapy is likely to be considered.

Increasingly, men with less advanced prostate cancer are also opting for hormonal therapy, either alone or in combination with radiation or surgery. When hormonal intervention is used to downsize the tumor prior to a primary treatment, it is referred to *neoadjuvant* therapy. Some men elect to undergo hormonal therapy instead of a primary therapy (radiation, surgery, or cryosurgery) because of individual health considerations, advanced age, fear of side effects, and so forth.

Hormonal therapy takes a variety of forms, both surgical (orchiectomy) and chemical, which rely on a common strategy for attacking the cancer. It has long been known that prostate cancer is to some extent dependent on and nourished by the male sex hormone, testosterone. This is one of a group of hormones known as androgens. The androgens are responsible for the masculine body changes associated with puberty: growth of body hair, increased muscle mass and genital size, and the deepening of a man's voice. Testosterone also regulates sexual desire, and influences moods and aggressiveness. Like other hormones, testosterone is a chemical released in the body through various biochemical mechanisms and carried in the bloodstream, where it can be detected by a blood test.

Since testosterone stimulates the growth of prostate cancer cells, depleting or ablating the body's testosterone tends to shrink the size of many tumors, specifically, those that are hormone-sensitive. The goal of hormonal therapy is to decrease the production of testosterone in the body, inhibiting the growth and progression of the cancer. These hormone-sensitive prostate cancers essentially are put into remission by the removal of the body's testosterone. In most cases, hormonal therapy will also significantly reduce pain and other symptoms of the disease when it has metastasized. Because hormonal therapy works against the body's production of the male hormones, it might be more accurately described as "anti-hormonal therapy."

Erectile dysfunction and loss of sexual desire are likely with almost every form of hormonal therapy. At least 95% of patients lose sexual desire and the ability to have an erection. Some of the newer hormonal agents discussed below have shown some improvement in maintaining sexual function.

While as many as 85% of prostate cancers are responsive to hormonal ablation, individual patient response to hormonal therapy varies widely. For those who initially respond to treatment, control of the disease may last from several months to many years. Two years is the average. As many as 10% of patients with metastatic disease survive for ten years or more, while more than 25% are still alive after five years. 80% of patients experience some relief of pain. However, in most cases, the cancer eventually becomes resistant to treatment, or *refractory,* and the patient will experience a relapse of the disease. This occurs because some of the cancer cells mutate and become *androgen-independent,* meaning that they are unaffected by male hormones. At this point, no form of hormonal therapy is likely to have a significant impact on the disease. Patients with androgen-independent prostate cancer (AIPC) can still resort to other forms of treatment, including at our institution a second line of androgen ablation therapy followed by chemotherapy and various chemical agents, which are often administered through clinical trials (see "What options are available once hormonal therapy stops working?").

In our practice we utilize a variety of regimes which may slow or stop prostate cancer growth, with chemotherapy considered as a last resort. These regimes for patients with advanced disease may include agents such as Casodex®, Dostinex®, Avodart®, estrogenic agents, Thalidomide, Cox-II inhibiters, agents which disrupt the IGF-1 pathway, Ketoconozole, and agents to improve bone integrity (biphosphonate), which not only counteract the adverse effects of hormones on bones, but which are also antineoplastic. Some of these agents are discussed in greater detail below.

How Does Hormonal Therapy Kill Cancer Cells?

Androgen deprivation causes what is known as programmed cell death, or *apoptosis,* which affects those cancer cells that are hormone-dependent. This results from a biochemical process referred to as *enzymatic DNA degradation.* Enzymes (often called "suicide enzymes") within the cell break down the genetic memory code and cause the cell to die. The mechanism of programmed cell death involves a long, complicated chain of biochemical events within each cell. Exactly how this process takes place is under continuing study by researchers who are seeking to develop more effective chemical agents to treat the disease. The challenge is to develop agents that kill the cancer cells without harming healthy prostate cells.

What is an Orchiectomy?

A bilateral orchiectomy involves the surgical removal of the testicles from the scrotum. This procedure is also known as surgical castration. Orchiectomy is one of several hormonal options for patients with late stage prostate cancer, though for most patients, this surgical procedure is the least appealing and is only rarely performed these days. Most men use injectable hormonal agents instead.

The testicles produce about 95 percent of the body's testosterone, and after their removal, a dramatic impact is often observed on the cancer, with a marked fall in the serum PSA level. Orchiectomy usually results in a retardation of the growth and spread of the cancer. Most tumors (both primary and metastases) shrink in size after a bilateral orchiectomy is performed. Patients also experience a significant alleviation of pain and other symptoms. In most cases, the benefits of orchiectomy will be temporary, and eventually the disease will reassert itself. Nevertheless, the procedure has been shown to stave off the symptomatic effects of the disease for many months or years.

Although the operation is minor and can be performed on an outpatient basis, using general or local anesthesia, most men find this surgery difficult to accept, even those patients who are no longer sexually active. The side effects associated with castrate testosterone levels vary considerably from patient to patient. Most men will experience loss of sexual desire and impotence following a bilateral orchiectomy. Hot flashes are a common side effect of the operation, affecting about one third of patients. Hot flashes involve a sudden rush of heat to the face, neck, upper chest, and back, lasting from a few seconds to an hour. These symptoms can be counteracted or ameliorated by various medications.

Orchiectomy may also cause mood changes, such as irritability or a loss of aggressiveness. Loss of muscle mass, weight gain, bone loss (osteopenia and osteoporosis) and changes in skin tone and hair growth are often late effects of treatment. Compared to other forms of hormonal therapy, a major disadvantage of bilateral orchiectomy is that it is irreversible.

What is Estrogen Therapy?

The administration of the female hormone, estrogen, inhibits the production of testosterone. Until recent years, this was the most common form of androgen deprivation therapy. When the pituitary gland in the brain detects the presence of female hormones, it stops production of male hormones by the testicles. Estrogenic compounds block the signal transmitted by the pituitary gland, known as luteinizing hormone (LH), which normally stimulates testosterone production. In the past, the most commonly prescribed form of estrogen was diethylstilbestrol, or DES®, taken orally. DES® is cheaper than most other hormone medications, but is no longer commonly prescribed because of the risk of blood clots. However, this risk is effectively countered by using blood thinners such as Coumadin. Estrogens have for the most part been replaced by LHRH agonists and anti-androgens, although estrogens remain an option when LHRH agonists and anti-androgens cease to work (see "What is LHRH therapy?").

Studies have shown DES® to be as effective as orchiectomy for temporarily halting the progression of prostate cancer. However, like orchiectomy, there are a number of side effects associated with estrogen therapy. These include fluid retention, breast enlargement and tenderness (gynecomastia), loss of sexual desire and erectile dysfunction, and rarely nausea and vomiting. Even more serious, estrogen therapy may result in severe circulatory or thrombotic problems, such as blood clots and stroke.

Aside from DES®, other drugs that have been used for estrogen therapy include Premarin® and ethinyl estradiol, which are medications also used by some women during menopause. In my practice, transdermal patches such as Estraderm®, Vivelle-Dot®, and Climara® are used to avoid metabolism of estrogen within the liver, and thereby reduce the risk of dangerous thrombotic side effects. For some men with advanced cancer who do not respond to other estrogen drugs, symptomatic relief may be achieved with polyestradiol phosphate (Stilphostrol®), which is given intravenously. Polyestradiol intramuscular (Estradurin®) may also be prescribed, administered by monthly injection. Another estrogen drug sometimes prescribed is estramustine phosphate (EMCYT®), which is taken orally, but it too carries the risk of serious side effects. PC SPES™ is an herbal form of hormonal therapy that was used until recently when the product was found to contain DES® and/or Coumadin and/or Indomethacin. This agent is therefore no longer available. Some men have used Prostasol with success similar to PC SPES™.

What is LHRH Therapy?

This form of hormonal therapy utilizes *leutinizing hormone releasing hormone* (LHRH) agonists (or analogs), a synthesized form of a natural brain hormone. LHRH agonists effectively shut down production of testicular testosterone, achieving the same effect as surgical removal of the testicles. LHRH agonists currently available in the U.S. include leuprolide (Lupron®, Viadur®, and Eligard®), goserelin (Zoladex®), and triptorelin (TRELSTAR®). LHRH agonists may be injected monthly or every 3, 4, or 12 months in the physician's office.

LHRH therapy has been a great benefit to those men who wish to avoid surgery. However, LHRH therapy is not without its disadvantages. The drugs are expensive, as they can cost $350 or more per month, which may be prohibitively high for some patients, although most insurance companies cover the cost in full (Medicare included). The side effects of LHRH agonists are similar to those associated with bilateral orchiectomy, namely hot flashes, some loss of libido, weight-gain, and in some cases erectile dysfuncton. Infrequent gastrointestinal side effects have been reported as well.

What is Combined Hormonal Therapy?

A "flare reaction" is observed when LHRH therapy is initiated, causing a brief rise or surge in testosterone level. The testosterone flare is accompanied by a rise in PSA and subsequent exacerbation of cancer symptoms, such as bone pain and urinary difficulties in some men. This initial phase typically lasts only a week or two. Small doses of estrogenic compounds, or *anti-androgens* such as flutamide (Eulexin®), bicalutamide (Casodex®), nilutamide (Nilandron®), and cyproterone acetate (Androcur®) may be administered 7 days prior to the initiation of LHRH therapy, as they act to block this flare phenomenon. This is a form of combined hormonal therapy, utilizing more than one hormonal agent. The anti-androgens prevent attachment of testosterone to prostate cells, and they are used to block the small percentage of testosterone produced by the adrenal glands.

The testosterone surge caused by LHRH therapy can be especially detrimental in men with localized prostate cancer, as it may promote cancer growth and potential dissemination. Unfortunately, all too many patients having localized prostate cancer receive LHRH agonists by their urologists without being given opposing agents such as estrogenic compounds or anti-androgens. This is an area of treatment about which urologists are often not as informed as oncologists, and do more harm than good.

The anti-androgen drugs may also cause side effects such as breast enlargement and nipple tenderness. These problems can be avoided by a short course of radiation therapy administered to the breast tissue. Others derive benefit from Arimidex or Tamoxifin. About 10% of men experience nausea and/or diarrhea when taking anti-androgens (especially with flutamide, though rarely with Casodex®). There is also some small risk of liver damage, and therefore, a blood test to check liver enzymes is usually given every three months.

Abarelix has been shown to induce castration-level testosterone without the temporary testosterone surge associated with drugs like Lupron®, Zoladex®, TRELSTAR®, and Viadur®. Often prescribed for patients with bone metastases, Abarelix also reduces pain and urinary symptoms. However, a small percentage of men (less than 5%) have serious allergic reactions to the drug. Abarelix is administered by injection every 2 weeks for the first month, and every 4 weeks thereafter. Patients are monitored for a half hour after being injected to be sure they do not show signs of allergic reaction.

What is Triple Hormonal Therapy?

This form of treatment combines the use of LHRH agonists (or, less commonly, orchiectomy) with an anti-androgen, and *5-alpha reductase inhibitor,* usually finasteride (Proscar®) or dutasteride (Avodart®). In the prostate gland, 5-alpha reductase is an enzyme that converts testosterone into a more potent growth stimulator or metabolite, dihydrotestosterone (DHT). This enzyme is blocked by the 5-alpha reductase inhibitors such as Proscar®, thus inhibiting the production of DHT. Many researchers now believe that the 5-alpha reductase inhibitors improve the efficacy of hormonal therapy.

A recent National Cancer Institute study has demonstrated that Proscar® actually prevents cancer for 25% of those patients taking the drug. That same study also reported that Proscar® encouraged more aggressive cancers in a small percentage of men, but that finding has since been refuted. It appears that tissue biopsies of those receiving Proscar® were falsely interpreted as being more aggressive.

Other recent studies have indicated that combination triple hormonal blockade is superior to other forms of hormonal therapy, extending the average period of remission by several months. In addition, the percentage of patients who respond to therapy is higher, and more men experience complete remission. However, clinical evaluation has been somewhat contradictory concerning the advantages of combination therapy over monotherapy (the use of a single hormonal regimen to suppress androgen production).

A modified combination therapy that uses flutamide (Eulexin® or Casodex®) with finasteride (Proscar® or Avodart®) allows many men to preserve potency while undergoing hormonal therapy. This limited combination of hormones (often referred to as Sequential Androgen Blockade, or SAB) can preserve quality of life, as neither of these drugs impact on sexual function to the extent that other hormonal agents do.

The mechanism of the SAB combination acts to block testosterone (and its more potent metabolite, DHT) on the cellular level of the tumor, while maintaining normal testosterone levels in the bloodstream, with the hope that the patient's sexual function will be preserved. However, with this approach there is a risk of breast enlargement and hypersensitivity of the nipples. These side effects can be counteracted by a short course of radiation delivered to the breast before starting therapy, or by administering drugs such as tamoxifen (Nolvadex®) or anastrozole (Arimidex®) to relieve the symptoms after they appear. A variation of this sequential approach substitutes bicalutamide (Casodex®) for flutamide to achieve the same end. Another approach using Casodex® at three times the typical daily dose (150 mg daily) achieves similar results without the dramatic impact on bone integrity and sexual dysfunction.

What is Intermittent Hormonal Therapy?

Intermittent hormonal therapy is a technique currently under investigation that offers the advantage of sparing patients side effects during intervals when they go off therapy. As previously noted, nearly all prostate cancers treated with androgen deprivation therapy become resistant to this treatment over a period of months or years. Some researchers, myself included, believe that constant androgen suppression may not be necessary, so they recommend intermittent (on-again, off-again) therapy.

At our institution, utilizing this approach, combination hormonal therapy (an LHRH agonist and an anti-androgen, plus or minus Proscar® or Avodart®) may be used for at least six months or more, and then stopped once the patient's PSA drops to an undetectable level. If the PSA level begins to rise to a predetermined value (e.g. 5 to 10), the drugs are started again. The off-phase of therapy can range from several months to several years or more, during which time patients can recover potency and quality of life. The resumption of the body's production of testosterone eventually restores normal blood testosterone levels and resolves most side effects caused by hormonal therapy; however, recovery time varies, and some patients are slow to recover their natural testosterone production.

How are Patients Monitored with Hormonal Therapy?

Patients are typically monitored every six months with a digital rectal exam, a PSA test, and chemistries to test for kidney function and liver function. If the PSA begins to rise, patients are given a bone scan once or twice a year to test for bone metastases. A blood test will also be used to measure the level of testosterone, to be sure it is within the castrate range and not fluctuating. With anti-androgens (Casodex®, flutamide), a blood test for liver enzymes is usually performed every 6 to 8 weeks and then every three months if stable. In addition, a number of medications are commonly prescribed to ensure bone integrity, in which case, calcium and magnesium levels require monitoring.

What Determines How Long Hormonal Therapy is Effective?

The benefits of hormonal therapy vary considerably from patient to patient. 10% of patients with advanced metastatic disease live longer than ten years. On the other hand, 10% live less than 6 months. Most patients fall somewhere in between, with 50% surviving three years or less.

Two factors appear to determine how long hormonal therapy is effective: the number of hormone-sensitive cells compared to the number of hormone-independent cells, and how fast the cancer is growing (the rate at which the cancer doubles in size). It is the hormone-independent cells that are ultimately fatal, and therefore, the rate at which they are growing is crucial. Research in the field is now focused on controlling these hormone-resistant cancer cells. If you are just beginning hormonal therapy today, it is entirely possible that new treatments will be available by the time hormones have ceased to work for you.

When Should Hormonal Therapy be Initiated?

During recent years there has been a growing enthusiasm for the early initiation of hormonal therapy, especially combination hormonal therapy. Early initiation means starting hormonal therapy before any symptoms of metastatic disease appear. Advocates of this approach point to those studies that indicate some degree of local control achieved with hormonal agents, slowing progression of the disease. It might appear to be common sense that because hormonal therapy lowers PSA, shrinks tumors and slows progression of the cancer, that it would also prolong life. But this may not be the case. Although the benefits of hormonal therapy for treating prostate cancer have been established, there is considerable controversy about how effective hormonal therapy may be at increasing survival.

Researchers remain divided on the optimal time to begin therapy, though recent studies favor early versus late initiation of hormonal therapy. The argument against early use of hormones rests on the fact that those who opt for early initiation will not be able to use hormonal therapy later when symptoms appear. By that time, the tumor may have become androgen-independent and refractory. After the beneficial effects of hormonal therapy have run their course, a patient's cancer may begin to grow again and eventually progress to what it would have been had hormonal therapy never been given. With this in mind, some doctors encourage men with advanced disease to embark on a course of watchful waiting (active surveillance), arguing that these patients should avoid side effects as long as possible since the treatment has not been shown to substantially prolong life. This conservative strategy calls for the use of hormone therapy only if and when symptoms appear.

Other researchers argue that men with metastatic disease yet smaller tumors and low Gleason scores (less aggressive cancer) might even be cured if treatment is started sooner because these patients have less cancer to begin with and slower growing cancer. As a tumor grows and becomes bulky, genetic changes may take place within the cancer cells that lead to androgen-independence; therefore, early treatment might offer some advantage for these patients by attacking the cancer before it becomes refractory. This point of view appears to be supported by a Mayo Clinic non-randomized study which indicated that patients with positive lymph nodes and low Gleason scores lived longer if they were treated hormonally before symptoms appeared.

Early stage (non-metastatic) patients should also be aware that the survival benefits of hormonal therapy have not been definitively established. Early initiation of hormonal therapy may indeed halt disease progression temporarily while these patients evaluate other primary treatment options. But a number of studies have demonstrated that early hormonal intervention prior to radical surgery does not reduce the risk of biochemical failure.

However, the early use of hormones appears to be more advantageous before undertaking radiation as a primary therapy. My own data does not demonstrate a strong advantage to utilizing hormones prior to radiation in patients having high risk features. Nonetheless, my patients who received hormones had far more aggressive tumors, and yet they fared similarly to those low risk patients who did not receive hormones. As the high risk group would have been expected to fare much worse, this would therefore support the use of hormones in this group. In addition, numerous multi-institutional studies both in the U.S. and abroad have demonstrated a benefit with the utilization of hormonal therapy prior to radiation.

It is clear that more men regardless of the stage of their cancer are choosing to initiate hormonal therapy early because of a perceived possibility of cure, or long-term remission. This option may seem appealing given the steady progress in the field and the likely development of new and more effective chemical agents in the near future. However, before making this choice, patients should fully investigate the potential side effects and changes in quality of life that can be anticipated with hormonal manipulation. Men who opt for early combination hormonal therapy should also keep in mind that the hormones are likely to stop working eventually. Regardless of the stage of cancer, patients should also consider lifestyle changes, including diet and nutrition (see Chapter 11: Diet and Nutrition Guidelines), homeopathics and agents like Celebrex® and Zyflamend®.

Hormonal therapy continues to be controversial because there are still so many unanswered questions in this area, and because doctors disagree about what the answers will turn out to be. The nature of this controversy makes it all the more important for patients to question their doctors carefully before embarking on treatment. Be sure your doctor has considerable experience with hormonal therapy, and find out what that experience has been with other patients of similar age and stage of cancer as your own. You should carefully discuss the pros and cons of each drug with your doctors and if you remain in doubt, by all means, obtain a second opinion. While the lack of definitive knowledge about hormonal therapy may be unsettling, each patient can still make an educated decision based on the possible benefits and risks associated with this form of treatment.

What Options are Available Once Hormonal Therapy Stops Working?

All combinations of hormonal therapy should be completely exhausted before further options are considered. For example, if the anti-androgen Eulexin® ceases to be effective, as indicated by a rising PSA, consideration might be given to changing to Casodex®, or another anti-androgen such as Nilandron® or Androcur®. There are a number of hormonal options available and new ones constantly being developed for FDA approval. After patients with advanced disease have exhausted all of these hormonal measures, alternative options may include chemotherapy and clinical trials that offer experimental treatments such as immunotherapy and vaccine therapies.

What are the Pros and Cons of the Various Hormonal Therapies?

Orchiectomy

Pros
1. Easy, quick, effective surgery
2. No ongoing drug therapy
3. Relatively inexpensive ($2000–$3500) compared to drugs

Cons
1. Psychological impact of castration
2. Does not supress adrenal androgens
3. Side effects of impotence, loss of libido, hot flashes
4. Irreversible procedure
5. Loss of bone integrity

Estrogen

Agents include DES®, Estraderm®, Climara®, Stilphostrol®, and Estradurin®

Pros

1. As effective as orchiectomy at achieving castrate-level testosterone
2. Relatively inexpensive compared to other hormonal drugs
3. Requires no surgery

Cons

1. Risk of cardiovascular problems (heart attack, stroke, blood clots)
2. Loss of sexual libido, hot flashes, fluid retention
3. Breast enlargement and/or tenderness
4. Does not supress adrenal androgens

LHRH Agonists

Agents include Lupron®, Zoladex®, TRELSTAR®, and Viadur®.

Pros

1. As effective as orchiectomy, without surgery
2. Low risk of cardiovascular problems
3. Fewer menopausal side effects than estrogen

Cons

1. Expensive ($4000 to $6000 annually)
2. Risk of tumor flare
3. High risk of erectile dysfunction and loss of libido
4. Hot flashes
5. Skin rash and irritation at injection site
6. Does not suppress adrenal androgens
7. Loss of bone integrity

Anti-androgens

Agents include Eulexin®, Casadex®, Nilandron®, and Androcur®.

Pros

1. Block adrenal androgens
2. Do not require surgery
3. Lower risk of testosterone flare caused by LHRH analogs
4. May increase survival in combination with orchiectomy, or LHRH analogs, or estrogen

Cons

1. Expensive ($4000 to $5000 annually)
2. Diarrhea (10%, especially with flutamide)
3. Small risk of liver toxicity (requiring monitor)
4. Some risk of breast enlargement and/or tenderness

What is Chemotherapy and How Effective is it in Treating Prostate Cancer?

Chemotherapy involves the use of potent toxins (*cytotoxic* agents) to treat cancer. These chemical substances are typically poisonous to both malignant and benign cells. Certain types of cancer such as leukemias and lymphomas are sensitive to relatively low doses of chemotherapy and can be cured by such drugs. Unfortunately, with the drugs that are currently available, chemotherapy is not usually effective in treating prostate cancer. Generally, greater than 25% of patients with metastatic prostate cancer respond to chemotherapy temporarily, though some of the more recent chemotherapy agents have shown somewhat better results. After administering the drugs, the tumors may shrink to some degree, but the shrinkage usually lasts only a few months, at which point the disease continues to progress.

The choice of whether or not to initiate chemotherapy is one that is made on a case by case basis by each patient in partnership with his doctor. Chemotherapy is typically limited to patients who do not respond or have become resistant to hormonal therapy. Since there is some chance that chemotherapy can bring about temporary remission of the cancer, many patients with advanced disease consider enrolling in clinical trials. These experimental studies provide data that will enable researchers to make better use of chemical agents in the future (See "How are clinical trials conducted and which patients are eligible?").

Some progress is being made by combining chemotherapy agents with other therapies to increase the likelihood that the cancer will shrink and to prolong the amount of time disease progression is interrupted. One recent study has reported promising 10-year results combining chemical agents (vinblastine, doxorubicin, and mitomycin) with radiation and hormonal therapy for the treatment of stage T3 (extracapsular extension) and N1 cancers (lymph node involvement). This study concludes, "The addition of chemotherapy to hormonal and radiation therapy is feasible and is accepted by most men when they are openly informed of their prognosis with conventional therapy" (Bagley CM et al: *Cancer. 2002 May 15; 94(10):2728-32)*. It should be noted that the patients in this study did not have distant metastases. It is not clear whether the results (greater than 70% biochemical disease-free progression) are superior to those achieved with hormonal therapy plus radiation alone, but as the authors point out, larger randomized studies are warranted.

What Chemical Agents are Currently Under Investigation?

Cytotoxic agents are the standard treatment for prostate cancer that does not respond to hormonal manipulation. There are numerous drugs in this class, and their side effects vary considerably. Attempts are being made to more effectively target cytotoxic agents to tumor sites, allowing for increased drug levels and cell death in cancerous tissues while minimizing toxicity for healthy tissues.

The following chemical agents and experimental therapies are among those being used for the treatment of advanced prostate cancer:

CYTADREN® (aminoglutethimide), usually administered in combination with hydrocortisone, selectively inhibits adrenal production of male hormones. Response rates in patients who have failed initial hormonal therapy are generally poor, although some patients have responded favorably to this therapy, with PSA levels falling 50% or more over periods of 2 to 6 months.

HYDROCORTISONE and other steroids fall into the category of endocrine therapies that work to decrease the receptivity of the cell's androgen receptor, thereby decreasing adrenal androgens. Steroids can cause excessive bone loss and usually require the use of bone supplements.

NIZORAL® (ketoconazole) is an antifungal agent that acts to inhibit male hormone production. Some positive results temporarily reducing PSA levels have been achieved using Nizoral® in patients whose cancers have become resistant to standard hormonal therapy. Hydrocortisone is always used simultaneously with Nizoral®.

VELBAN (vinblastine) is a chemotherapy drug being studied in combination with other agents such as the estrogenic compound, estramustine phosphate (Emcyt®), for treating hormone-refractory prostate cancer. Clinical trials with this combination have reported temporary PSA decreases of 50% or more in a significant number of patients.

PROGESTINS such as hydroxyprogesterone caproate, megestrol acetate, and medrogestone, inhibit testosterone production, and have resulted in limited, temporary responses in some patients. These drugs are being studied in combination with other chemotherapy agents in a number of ongoing clinical trials.

TAXANES such as Taxotere® (docetaxel) and Taxol® (paclitaxel) are a class of drugs that have been used in treating breast and ovarian cancers as well as prostate cancer since the 1990s. These and similar drugs are showing increasing efficacy in temporarily improving quality of life for patients with metastatic disease. Many researchers believe this type of chemotherapy will give way to or complement more promising immunologic and angiogenesis therapies (see below).

SURAMIN is a growth factor inhibiting agent under investigation for the treatment of hormone-refractory prostate cancer. Early results were promising, with response rates as high as 70%, but subsequent randomized tests have been less impressive with only about 20% of patients showing reduced PSA levels over a period of months and a reduction in pain associated with bone metastases. The National Cancer Institute is currently sponsoring clinical trials combining suramin with Cytadren®.

APTOSYN® (exisulind) is a drug that has shown some promise in clinical trials and is undergoing further testing. It acts by directing cancerous tissue to undergo programmed cell death (apoptosis) without damaging healthy tissue. One study at Columbia University evaluated the effects of Aptosyn® on locally recurrent prostatectomy patients and found the drug slowed PSA doubling time, suggesting that the initiation of hormonal therapy might be delayed for these patients. Other trials are now underway combining Aptosyn® with Taxotere® for the treatment of hormone-refractory prostate cancer.

PROVENGE® is an immunologic or "vaccine" therapy that directs the body's immune system to destroy cancer cells. Trials are currently underway to test a number of immunologic therapies on patients with hormone-refractory prostate cancer. This approach takes advantage of the fact that the body has cells that are programmed to destroy foreign targets (antigens). Vaccine therapies treat cancer as if it were a foreign agent invading the body, something analogous to a bacterial infection. The goal of researchers is to stimulate the patient's immune system with antigens that mimic the antigens of the cancer cell, thereby causing the immune system to attack the cancer.

ATRASENTAN® is an agent known as an ET *receptor antagonist,* which acts to block a prostate cancer cell product (Endothelin-1 or ET-1) that stimulates *osteoblastic metastases* (bone lesions). ET-1 also acts to constrict blood vessels (vasoconstriction) that may account for bone pain in patients with metastatic cancer. Early results with Atrasentan have shown some promise in slowing disease progression, especially in patients with skeletal metastases.

COX-II INHIBITORS are a class of drugs that include Celebrex®, widely used as an arthritis medication. The Cox-II inhibitors have shown promise in clinical trials for treating a number of genitourinary cancers, including prostate cancer. Cox-II inhibitors relieve pain, inflammation, and swelling by blocking the body's production of an enzyme called Cox-II. A number of studies are underway to evaluate the effectiveness of these drugs in slowing or preventing the progression of prostate cancer. An herbal Cox-II inhibitor, Zyflamend, is currently available.

ANGIOSTATIN and ENDOSTATIN are agents that act on the molecular level to inhibit the growth of blood vessels that allow tumors to grow and metastasize. In order for tumors to grow, they require nutrients supplied through a network of capillaries. The process by which tumors establish this network of blood vessels is known as *angiogenesis*. Agents like angiostatin and endostatin that interfere with angiogenesis are being tested both as single agents and in combination with other therapies in the hope that such strategies can destroy both androgen-dependent and androgen-independent tumors.

THALIDOMIDE is another agent that acts as an angiogenesis inhibitor, and it may also inhibit COX-II induction. There has been a resurgence of interest in Thalidomide since the 1960s when it was found to cause birth defects. A number of clinical trials have shown promising results in treating androgen-independent prostate cancer. One study of Thalidomide administered as sole agent showed a PSA decline of 50% or more in 18% of patients, and a PSA decline of 40% or more in 27% of patients (Figg W.D. et al, *Clinical Cancer Research, July 2001, Vol. 7, 1888-1893)*. Thalidomide is also being studied in combination with various cytotoxic chemotherapy agents.

ONCOLYTIC VIRUSES are man-made anti-cancer agents produced through genetic engineering. Viruses can be used to transfer genes into a cancer cell. Genetic manipulation allows these viruses to selectively destroy cancer cells by inducing cell death, or *lysis*. There are a number of specific oncolytic viruses under investigation, with names like Cell Genesys Viruses CG7060 and CG7870, Reolysin®, and ONYX-15.

Another strategy utilizing viruses has been to engineer viral strains that can actually restore cancer cells to normal by infusing corrective genetic information, replacing defective genes and thereby rectifying the uncontrolled cell growth that is characteristic of malignant cells. Gene therapy also targets specific genes or proteins such as bcl-2 or p-53, which are involved with the process of programmed cell death.

ANTISENSE THERAPY is a type of gene therapy that involves the use of synthetic DNA and RNA segments called *oligonucleotides* to stop or interrupt the production of cancer-related proteins. Antisense compounds block the transmission of genetic information between the nucleus and protein production sites within the cell, inhibiting genes that are responsible for cancer growth and for resistance to drug therapies. Antisense olignonucleotides targeting the bcl-2 protein has been shown to induce apoptosis and enhance chemosensitivity when used in combination with agents like paclitaxel (Taxol®).

New anti-cancer agents are continuously under development. Several are not mentioned here because research findings into the efficacy of the agents have yet to be made public. With our increasing knowledge regarding the molecular and cellular mechanisms by which prostate cancer progresses, it is very likely that new agents with improved therapeutic potential will be available in the near future.

How are Clinical Trials Conducted and Which Patients are Eligible?

When traditional avenues of treatment are exhausted, men with advanced disease may wish to consider participating in a clinical trial. Trials generally test new treatments and compare them with traditional therapies. They are usually not undertaken as a primary treatment, but may be appropriate for patients with limited therapeutic options. The purpose of a trial is to benefit the patient, whether by prolonging life, improving quality of life, or alleviating pain. If you are considering enrolling in a clinical trial, you should carefully investigate the proposed treatment to be sure you meet the eligibility requirements, as eligibility varies from program to program.

Clinical trials are carried out in three phases. Phase I trials are used to determine doses and toxicity of new drugs and therapies. After the optimal dose is determined, a Phase II trial will be carried out with a limited number of patients to evaluate the effectiveness of the drug or therapy. Before a new drug or therapy becomes FDA-approved, a Phase III trial will be conducted to compare the effectiveness of the newly developed treatment to currently available treatments within a larger population.

If you decide to pursue a clinical trial, you will want to find out whether you are going to receive the new drug or therapy, or instead be part of a double-blind study in which a control or placebo group does not receive the new medication or therapy. If patients fail to receive a benefit from a drug because they are part of a placebo group, they are usually given the drug at the end of the trial. Patients are advised not to give up the opportunity for an established treatment of known effectiveness in favor of a clinical trial in which the efficacy of the new therapy is unknown.

Clinical trials are often conducted by comprehensive medical centers, which develop and test new therapies and therapeutic agents. Trials are also organized by pharmaceutical companies in response to an FDA request to establish the value and safety of a particular drug before it can be marketed. Patients may wish to contact one or more of the comprehensive medical centers located in their area. In the Northeast, some of the premier medical centers include Memorial Sloan-Kettering, Johns Hopkins, Dana Farber, Columbia, the National Cancer Institute (N.C.I.). Baylor University and M.D. Anderson are in the south, and the University of Michigan is in the Midwest. West coast centers include UCLA and the University of California in San Francisco. For further information on clinical trials, patients are encouraged to contact the National Cancer Institute's Cancer Information Service at 1-800-4-CANCER, or their Web site: http://cis.nci.nih.gov/

What Therapies Can Alleviate Pain for Patients with Advanced Cancer?

Patients should never hesitate to discuss pain and other quality of life concerns with their doctors. There are a number of effective therapies for relieving pain and most other symptoms associated with prostate cancer and the side effects of treatment. Alleviating pain will allow you not only to concentrate and to make decisions about your treatment, but will also enable you to continue to enjoy life and the things that matter most to you.

When properly prescribed, pain medications including narcotic drugs (opioids) can be very effective. External radiation therapy is utilized as a palliative therapy to relieve pain in patients with metastatic disease. Other forms of radiation are also used to alleviate pain. Samarium-153 (Quadramet®) and Strontium-89 Chloride (Metastron®) are FDA-approved radio-pharmaceuticals administered by injection. They go directly to the sites of metastatic bone disease to relieve pain symptoms. A single injection of either of these radioisotopes may alleviate pain for three to six months, after which, the patient can receive repeat injections at intervals of 90 days or more when medically appropriate.

Bisphosphonate compounds, such as Actonel®, Fosamax®, Boniva®, and Aredia®, are drugs that can relieve pain caused by cancer that has metastasized to the bones and may also retard the growth of these metastases. Zoledronic acid (Zometa®) was the first bisphosphonate approved for use in bone metastases caused by prostate cancer. Other bisphosphonates have been approved for other medical uses, and some doctors prescribe them "off label" (a drug prescribed to treat a condition for which it has not been FDA approved) to treat prostate cancer. These substances have an anti-cancer effect and also help prevent or correct bone loss (osteopenia and osteoporosis), which is an unwanted complication of hormonal therapy.

CHAPTER NINE

THE FACTS: PROSTATE CANCER TREATMENT OPTION SUMMARIES

A comprehensive list comparing "The Facts" about treatment options for prostate cancer was published recently by the Dattoli Cancer Center & Brachytherapy Research Institute. This fact sheet premiered September 6, 2008 at the Prostate Cancer Research Institute's annual international conference in Los Angeles. Adapted from that document, the listing below runs from Surgery to Watchful Waiting, and includes a description of the pros, cons and information on published success rates of the various treatment options currently available in the US.

The original "Facts" list on treatment options is available from the Dattoli Cancer Center (see Appendix, "Where to Get Help"), or it can be downloaded as an Adobe PDF file from Dattoli Cancer Center website: www.dattoli.com.

As you consider this treatment option tool, keep in mind that the challenge of treatment remains how to kill the cancer cells without permanently damaging the critical structures that surround the prostate gland. As we have seen in earlier chapters, depending on the stage of the disease when diagnosed and the experience level of the treating physician, treatment has too often left the man with erectile dysfunction and/or incontinence. Newer therapies are designed to protect these functions and quality of life while destroying the malignant prostate cancer cells, but many have not yet proven their effectiveness. As you conduct your own research and consult with your doctor, you will need to use your own best judgment based on the facts, the specifics of your case and your own personal needs.

Surgical Treatments

In the past, surgery was considered the Gold Standard treatment for prostate cancer, but today, with virtually no advantages and many disadvantages compared to other forms of treatment, for many doctors, surgery has increasingly fallen into disfavor.

Radical Prostatectomy

Description: Surgical removal of the bulk of the gland by incisions either retropubic or perineal.

Pros: Physically removes the tumor from the body

Cons: Most aggressive surgery to be performed on the patient's body but least aggressive in treating the cancer. Often leaves microscopic cancer cells behind.

Published Results: Results have been reported for many years, as this was the only treatment for decades.

References: Moule, J Urol,Vol 163, 2000, showing "30,000 men per year will develop recurrence after radical prostatectomy."

Robotic "da Vinci" Laparoscopy

Description: Uses "sophisticated" robotic equipment to remove gland tissue through small openings in the abdomen.

Pros: Possibly easier to tolerate than open surgery.

Cons: The robotic approach is still surgery, with surgery's failings as a curative treatment. Success is very dependent on operator's level of experience and expertise.

Published Results: Recent studies report a 3-fold increase in the failure rate at only 6 months.

Reference: Blute, Michael L., Mayo Clinic, J Clin Onc, Vol 26, No 14, May 10, 2008: "Patients have been led to believe that hospital and recovery times are shorter and outcomes are better, but study has shown this expectation not to be the case."

Radiation Treatments

There are many types of radiation and delivery systems. The advantages of radiation therapy include no cutting, no blood loss, and much lower risk of infection than surgery. Potential drawbacks are eliminated by the experience and expertise of physicians with a proven track record.

Brachytherapy

Implanting radioactive sources (seeds, pellets) directly into the tumor. The ability to place the radiation source exactly at the site of the cancer is an advantage; however, results are dependant on the skill of the brachytherapist to place the seeds appropriately. Many studies have been published over the past 10 years, including Dattoli, Wallner, Merrick, Blasko and Sharkey.

PALLADIUM-103

Description: Isotope with short half-life and steep dose fall-off.

Pros: Radiation effects diminish by 50% every 17 days; seeds rarely migrate by design.

Cons: None noted.

Published Results: Numerous long term studies (Dattoli, Wallner, Merrick, and Blasko, among others).

Reference: Dattoli, et al, Long-term prostate cancer control using palladium-103 brachytherapy and external beam radiotherapy in patients with a high likelihood of extracapsular cancer extension; Urology. 2007 Feb;69(2):334-7.

IODINE-125

Description: Isotope with longer half-life and broader dose dispersion to patient, family members, and pets.

Pros: None noted.

Cons: The shape of iodine seeds can cause them to migrate from the target.

Published Results: Numerous, including comparisons to PD-103.

Reference: Wallner, The Cancer Journal, 2002,8(1):67-73.

IRIDIUM-192 (High Dose Rate: HDR)

Description: Using Iridium-192, highly penetrating, potentially damaging isotope.

Pros: Use of new microprocessors.

Cons: Penetrating nature of Iridium causes significant radiation exposure to entire body.

Published Results: Numerous.

Reference: Int J Rad Onc Biol/Phy,Vol 65 No 1, 2006, showing large field radiation exposure with HDR.

EBRT

Description: External Beam Radiation uses fractionated photon doses.

Pros: Early version of technology; noninvasive modality.

Cons: Now outdated technology.

Published Results: Outdated studies.

IMRT

Description: Intensity Modulated Radiation Therapy with photons.

Pros: More controlled and accurate version of EBRT (and 3D-Conformal Radiation Therapy).

Cons: Now "old" technology: the early generation of this modality has already been surpassed.

Published Results: Outdated studies.

Reference: Zelefsky, et al, J Urol, 166, 2001

4D-IG IMRT

Description: Four-Dimension Image-Guided IMRT with photons.

Pros: With DART (Dynamic Adaptive RT) the most exquisite control of beams.

Cons: Very few medical centers offer this level of technology.

Published Results: Evolutionary, in progress 2009.

Proton Therapy

Description: Uses protons to kill cancer cells.

Pros: Excellent treatment for tiny tumors of the eyes and brain. Advantages become disadvantages when treating large areas such as the prostate.

Cons: Risks of radiation "scatter"; not effective for large areas (prostate); risk of secondary tumors from proton by-product (neutrons). Not widely available.

Published Results: Clinical studies do not show proton therapy to be as safe and effective as the most sophisticated forms of photon radiation.

Reference: Hall, et al, Int J Onc, Vol 65, No 1,2006: "When compared to photons, a 10-fold increased total-body dose delivered to patient by neutrons."

Neutron Therapy

Description: Uses neutrons to kill cancer cells.

Pros: Theoretically, neutrons might be effective for treating cancers resistant to photon radiation.

Cons: Much less accurate than other forms of radiation. Any contact of the neutron beam with healthy tissue can cause severe damage, so there is an unacceptably high incidence of serious side effects. Not widely available.

Published Results: Neutron therapy is still experimental and studies do not show it to be as safe and effective as the most sophisticated forms of photon radiation. With the ability of photons to reach higher doses than ever before as a result of technological advances (i.e., 4D IG-IMRT with DART, and brachytherapy), the concept of tumors being resistant to photons has taken on less and less importance in recent years.

References: Lindsley, K.L., et al, Fast neutrons in prostatic adenocarcinomas: worldwide clinical experience; Recent Results Cancer Res. 1998;150:125-36. Santanam L., Intensity modulated neutron radiotherapy for the treatment of adenocarcinoma of the prostate; Int J Radiat Oncol Biol Phys. 2007 Aug 1;68(5):1546-56.

Cyberknife

Description: The fancy name actually refers to a method of radiation delivery; "hypo-fractionated" dose delivery (fewer sessions but higher doses of photon radiation).

Pros: Treatment usually delivered in only 5 fractions.

Cons: Studies reveal significant complications including high incidence of urethral/rectal fistula, bladder damage, ulcerations, bone necrosis.

Published Results: No long-term results published (should be reserved for non-curative cases; patients who will not live long enough to suffer harsh complications).

Reference: Prostate Cancer blog entry (www.nyprosate.blogspot.com), Dr. Louis Potters, 2/14/07.

Tomotherapy

Description: CT-guided IMRT ("new"), using photons.

Pros: In theory, delivers radiation in helical pattern; best used for small targets.

Cons: Reported problems with consistent movement of patient couch.

Published Results: Yes, but no long term results.

Note: There is a class action lawsuit against the manufacturer for alleged insider stock infractions.

Combination Therapy

Description: Using two or more types of radiation, sometimes with hormones, to defeat cancer.

Pros: Cancers of all sites proven to respond best to multiple modalities; temporary side effects.

Cons: Success dependent on expertise of practitioner, staff, costly equipment.

Published Results: Longest published survival rates: 16 years, using IMRT with PD-103 brachytherapy.

Reference: Dattoli, Cancer, Vol 110, No 3, 08/07 pp 551-555.

Other Treatment Options

Cryotherapy (aka Cryoablation and Cryosurgery)

Description: As primary treatment, uses the process of freezing and thawing to destroy cancer cells.

Pros: No cutting; performed on outpatient basis.

Cons: Highest risk of permanent impotence and high rate of incontinence. Cancers typically return. Lack of long-term data.

Published Results: Few long term studies (not recommended for cases where cancer is known or suspected to have spread).

Reference: Long, Bahn, Lee Urol, 57:518-523, 2001

HIFU (High Intensity Focused Ultrasound)

Description: Uses focused sound waves from a rectal probe to ablate cancer cells. Waves heat the target area to destroy tissue; several hour-long sessions required.

Pros: No cutting; non-ionizing (treatment can be repeated).

Cons: Just another form of "hypothermia" (heat therapy) used over 50 years ago and abandoned as cancers virtually always return with aggression.

Published Results: Few long term studies (not recommended for cases where cancer is known or suspected to have spread).

Reference: Misrai, World J Onc, Springer-Verlag 2008: 43.7% experienced biochemical recurrence in less than 5 years.

Hormonal Therapy

Description: Uses various types of hormones to decrease production of testosterone to inhibit growth and progress of cancer. Hormonal therapy is often used when treating advanced disease (metastatic cancer). It is also used in conjunction with radiation therapy as a primary treatment for early stage disease.

Pros: Easy oral or injection treatment.

Cons: Side-effects: impotence and menopause like symptoms (hot flashes, fragile bones, enlarged painful breasts). Cancers become resistant. Expensive.

Published Results: Many studies indicate hormonal therapy is appropriate only when all other options have been expended when treating advanced disease.

Reference: Keating, J Clin Onc, Vol 24, No 27: 4448-4454, examining hormonal therapy's unwelcome side-effects, including treatment-related diabetes and cardiovascular disease.

Watchful Waiting

Description: No treatment but periodic retesting to assess disease progression.

Pros: Easier to tolerate as long as cancer does not spread.

Cons: Can produce the anxiety of "watchful worrying."

Published Results: Controversial studies on survival benefits, but recommended for elderly with less than 5 years life expectancy.

References: Lancet Onc., 2008 May 9(5): 407-9, showing "4-fold increase in mortality without treatment."

PART THREE

BY JENNIFER CASH, ARNP, MS, OCN®

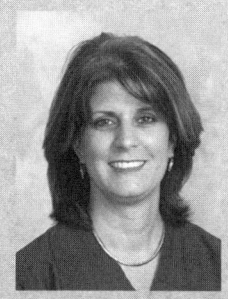

In my capacity as an Advanced Registered Nurse Practitioner (ARNP), I am often the first care provider to have contact with patients prior to treatment. We nurses, as frontline caregivers, are in a unique position to guide patients with support and reassurance throughout their course of treatment and recovery. Through education about the disease process, the treatment procedure and its associated side effects, we strive to deliver a high quality of care with a holistic approach that takes into account the physical, emotional and mental health of our patients.

POST-TREATMENT CARE AND LIFESTYLE CHANGES

As a member of a brachytherapy and radiation oncology team, I routinely counsel patients as well as their families before, during and after treatment. In the pages that follow, part of my discussion of side effects and quality of life concerns is directed to those patients undergoing radiation therapy. This group of patients now represents the majority of those being treated for localized prostate cancer. However, many of the specific comments and guidelines offered here also apply to surgical patients and others who may experience treatment-related side effects such as erectile dysfunction or incontinence.

CHAPTER TEN

COPING WITH SIDE EFFECTS

As Dr. Dattoli indicated in his discussion, all of the primary, curative treatments for prostate cancer carry some risk of temporary and long-term side effects. Even men who are successfully treated may find their triumph over the disease eclipsed by the subsequent complications of their treatment. The most common and distressing complications are incontinence and erectile dysfunction. Fortunately, there are a variety of therapies available to help patients cope with these untoward side effects. In addition, there are a number of remedies to reduce or ameliorate the short term side effects commonly experienced by men who undergo brachytherapy and external radiation therapy.

Post-implant Side Effects

While brachytherapy carries the lowest risk of permanent complications, most seed implant patients experience short term side effects such as urethral irritation, which may include frequency, urgency, decreased flow of the urine stream, pain upon urination (dysuria) and getting up at night to urinate (nocturia). Few patients experience urinary obstruction and/or long term dysuria. Rectal symptoms are uncommon; however, some patients do experience soft stools and/or increased frequency of bowel movements. Perineal discomfort immediately following treatment is usually minimal and easily remedied by oral steroidal and non-steroidal anti-inflammatory agents and mild analgesics. Sitz baths (sitting in warm water for 15 to 20 minutes) or ice packs may also be used to treat rectal or perineal discomfort. Some patients may also experience painful ejaculations that resolve with time.

The duration of urinary and rectal side effects is shorter with palladium implants than with iodine implants because of palladium's shorter half-life. Immediate postoperative urinary side effects may occur 7 to 10 days after the brachytherapy procedure. With Pd-103, symptoms usually peak in severity within 2 to 4 weeks, but they may persist at a higher level for 2 to 3 months. With I-125, these same symptoms may last 10 to 12 months. There are many factors that may influence the duration of urinary symptoms: having a history of prostatitis, enlarged prostate gland, dietary intake, and non-compliance with prescribed medications. These are routinely managed as indicated. *It should be also noted that patients who have received IMRT prior to brachytherapy, do not experience any significant increase in the temporary side effects associated with implantation.*

At our institution, after a patient is discharged following brachytherapy, a number of medications are commonly prescribed. These include the following:

> An anti-inflammatory to help reduce swelling of the prostate. Typically, a steroid anti-inflammatory will be used for several days, and thereafter a non-steroidal anti-inflammatory such as ibuprofen.

> An over-the-counter medication like Pepcid® AC may be used with the anti-inflammatory to prevent stomach upset.

> An antibiotic is routinely prescribed to prevent infection in the post-operative period.

> An alpha-blocker such as Flomax®, Uroxatral®, Hytrin® or Cardura® is prescribed to aid the flow of urination. This is the most important medication for the treatment of urinary symptoms. Patients usually continue using an alpha-blocker for several weeks to several months, depending on the duration of symptoms.

> Hydrocortisone suppositories are used as a preventative medication to ameliorate any rectal irritation that may result from the ultrasound rectal probe used during the seeding procedure, or from irritation caused by the radiation, or from pre-existing hemorrhoids.

➤ Over-the-counter medications such as Azo Standard® or Azo Cran-berry®, sodium bicarbonate tablets, or Prelief® may be used to help with any urinary burning or discomfort.

➤ Over-the-counter preparations such as Metamucil or Citracel may be used for constipation or looseness of the bowels.

It should also be noted that radiation patients are advised to avoid all antioxidant supplements such as Vitamins A, C, E, beta carotene and sele-nium, as these may have an opposing action to the radiation treatment. For long term nutritional guidelines following treatment and beyond this three month interval, see Chapter Eleven: Diet and Nutrition Guidelines.

Common Bladder Irritants Post-Seeding

After brachytherapy, the following foods may cause painful or more fre-quent urination. Some men can tolerate limited amounts of these foods, while other men cannot. 6 to 8 weeks after seeding, patients can try to slowly reintroduce these foods into their diets. Keep in mind that while this may seem to be an exhaustive listing, patients may find they are sensitive other foods as well.

The most common irritants are:

➤ Coffee (Reg. or de-caf)
➤ Tea (Reg. or de-caf)
➤ Carbonated beverages
➤ Citrus fruit drinks
➤ Alcohol
➤ Spicy or hot foods
➤ Tomatoes
➤ Peppers

➤ Sugar
➤ Honey
➤ Lemon Juice
➤ Lima Beans
➤ Yogurt
➤ Sugar
➤ Honey

Other foods that may cause urinary problems include the following:

➤ Apricots
➤ Avocados
➤ Bananas
➤ Brewers Yeast
➤ Cantaloupe
➤ Cheese (aged)

➤ Chicken Livers
➤ Chilies
➤ Citrus Fruits/Juices (especially with fortified Vitamin C)
➤ Corn Syrup
➤ Fava Beans

- Foods High In Potassium
- Grapes
- Honey
- Lima Beans
- Milk Products
- Mayonnaise
- Nuts (in general)
- Nutrasweet
- Onions
- Peaches
- Pineapple
- Plums
- Rye Bread
- Saccharine
- Sour Cream
- Soy Sauce
- Spicy Foods
- Strawberries
- Sugar
- Vinegar
- Vitamins buffered with Aspirate
- Yogurt

Milder Substitutes

The following milder foods can be substituted for those on the previous list of common bladder irritants. These items should be used sparingly and on a limited basis for the first 6 to 8 weeks after treatment. Remember, each individual is different, so these foods should be introduced slowly into the patient's diet in order to gauge his reaction.

- Almonds
- Apple–small
- Blueberries
- Cashews
- Carob
- Fish
- French Sauternes
- Frozen Yogurt
- Garlic
- Imitation Sour Cream
- Melons
- Onions–cooked
- Pears
- Pine Nuts
- Poultry
- Processed Cheeses (not aged)
- Shallots
- Spring Water
- Zest of Oranges or Limes

Urinary Incontinence

Urinary incontinence (involuntary urine leakage or dribbling) is a common side effect after radical surgery, however, it also affects a very small percentage of men treated with radiation. Incontinence may be temporary but it is rarely permanent. It is also influenced by previous surgeries of the bowel, bladder and prostate (TURP).

Incontinence is more than a physical disorder. If left untreated or managed improperly after surgery, it can affect quality of life. If you are a patient having difficulty with urinary control, you may feel embarrassed about discussing the problem, but keep in mind that you are not alone and there are effective remedies. You may harbor feelings of anxiety or anger, or you may feel isolated because of the condition. Fear of having an accident may prevent you from taking part in normal activities. By reporting the problem to your doctor, he can evaluate the nature and extent of the condition and recommend an appropriate treatment option or options. These may include one or more of the following:

Medications

If the bladder outlet muscle is unstable, drugs such as Detrol®, Ditropan®, Oxytrol™, Enablex® and Vesicare® may also be used to relax the bladder and reduce the pressure it exerts on stored urine, thereby minimizing leakage.

Kegel exercises

Special exercises are another technique often used to treat incontinence. Kegel exercises involve alternate tightening and relaxing of the sphincter muscles at the base of the pelvis, as if trying to hold in urine. These exercises can help restore lost urinary control for many men. A study in 2003 at the Kaiser Permanente Medical Center in Los Angeles found that surgical patients who did Kegel exercises regained control of continence faster than men who didn't exercise. Biofeedback may also be used to train and strengthen the muscles that control urination.

Erectile Dysfunction (ED)

Erectile dysfunction is a possible outcome of any form of treatment for prostate cancer, although there is a higher risk with radical surgery and cryosurgery than with seed implants and IMRT. Even patients who undergo nerve-sparing prostatectomies are quite likely to experience impaired sexual function. ED is also a common side effect in men who have had orchiectomies and those who are prescribed hormonal agents.

Men who are in their later years and no longer sexually active are not likely to be concerned about this complication. But most patients who are still sexually active before treatment will be anxious to take some action to restore any loss of ability to achieve an erection. There is no simple test for erectile dysfunction. The only way for a doctor to know that a sexual problem exists is through statements from the patient himself. To complicate matters, sexual problems may have both psychological and physical causes. Sometimes merely anticipating erectile problems after treatment will cause men to experience a loss of normal erectile function. Stress, anxiety and depression can also contribute to the problem. More recently, smoking has been found to be a profound contributor to erectile dysfunction, as are obesity and diabetes.

Referral for a diagnostic analysis is usually the first step in treating potency problems. This entails detailed questioning to ascertain the nature of the problem. If the ability to achieve an erection varies depending on the time or circumstances, then at least part of the problem is likely to be psychological and may be treated through counseling. To determine if there is a physical basis for the problem, a doctor may perform tests to measure blood pressure and pulse in the penis. These may indicate that circulation problems are impairing the patient's ability to have an erection. A blood test may also be used to check the level of male hormones. Because many men experience erections during sleep, a sleep laboratory evaluation is sometimes performed. Normal erections experienced during sleep indicate that the problem does not have a physical basis.

In many cases, however, a physical cause for erectile dysfunction will be found. There are several potential physical causes. Surgery can sever the nerves or proximal penile tissue that control erection. Vascular damage may be another cause of sexual dysfunction after radiation therapy, as damage to the blood vessels can reduce the blood flow to the penis needed to achieve an erection. Certain medications, such as those used to treat high blood pressure, diabetes and depression, may also contribute to erectile problems.

A number of treatment options are available for men suffering from erectile dysfunction. These include the following:

Phosphodiesterase inhibitors. Drugs such as sildenafil (Viagra®), vardenafil (Levitra®), and tadalafil (Cialis®) have been very effective in helping to restore erectile function after treatment. With brachytherapy and IMRT, more than 90% of men who were sexually active prior to treatment are able to retain sexual function post-implant. With surgical patients, Viagra® is significantly less effective and will not work for men who have had both neurovascular bundles removed or damaged. According to one study, erectile function was preserved in 71% of patients undergoing bilateral nerve-sparing RP, 50% of patients undergoing unilateral RP, and 15% of those men who had RPs without utilizing the nerve-sparing procedure (Zippe CD et al, Urology 55: 241-245. 2000).

Viagra® and similar drugs increase blood flow to the penis to help achieve and maintain a satisfactory erection. These drugs only work when a man is sexually stimulated, and do not increase sexual desire (libido). They can cause side effects including headaches, flushing, indigestion, light sensitivity and other visual problems, and runny or stuffy nose. Most of these side effects are mild and short-lived, however, in some cases more serious problems can occur. Patients who experience prolonged erections (four hours or more) should seek medical attention immediately.

Interactions with other drugs are also possible, so be sure your doctor knows what medications you are taking. Drugs that contain nitrates, which are often used for treating heart disease, can interact with these potency drugs to cause very low blood pressure, a potentially fatal complication. The use of Viagra®, Levitra® and Cialis® should be used with caution by patients who are taking alpha blockers (Flomax®, Hytrin®, Cardura®, Minipress®, Uroxatral®), as the interaction with these medications may cause a similar drop in blood pressure. Before taking any of these potency drugs, you should inform your doctor if you have a history of heart problems, low or high blood pressure, a history of stroke, kidney or liver problems, stomach ulcer, blood cell abnormalities, Peyronie's disease, or any other significant health problem.

Injections. A variety of other drugs can be used to treat erectile dysfunction. Papaverine, Phentolamine, and Prostaglandin E1 are drugs used to relax muscles and increase the blood supplied to the penis. Injections are made directly into the penis, initially by the physician and later by the patient himself. Although many men find the idea of penile injections unpleasant, they cause only minimal discomfort.

Men uncomfortable with needles can get a simple device that automatically injects medication with the press of a button. Prostaglandin E1 can also be applied to the surface of the penis or inserted in the form of a urethral pellet (Muse®), thereby eliminating the need for injections.

Penile Implants. Intrapenile prosthetic devices can be a satisfactory solution for men who wish to continue having intercourse. A penile prosthesis is surgically inserted inside the shaft of the penis. The penile implants currently available fall into two basic categories: those that are inflatable and those that are semi-rigid. The advantages and disadvantages of each type of prosthesis should be discussed by the patient and his physician. Men should also include their partners in decisions about implants and other erectile aids.

Vacuum Devices. These non-surgical devices use vacuum suction and penile constriction to assist blood flow into the penis, causing an erection. They consist of a plastic cylinder placed over the penis and a hand-held pump to draw air from the cylinder. Once an erection is achieved, an elastic band is placed around the base of the penis to maintain erection. Although less popular than injections or implant devices, these devices are often effective and have the advantage of being non-invasive.

Surgical Treatment. For those patients who suffer from vascular blockage that does not respond to other treatments, an experimental surgical procedure may be performed. An artery that usually supplies blood to the stomach is rerouted by the surgeon and connected to blood vessels inside the penis. Results with this procedure so far have been not been very successful.

Over the Counter Products. There are also over the counter products to improve sexual perfomance. Supplements that may help include zinc, L-Arginine, Yohimbe, Chrysin, Avena Sativa, stinging nettles, Tribulus, and Muira Pauma. It should be noted that testosterone enhancers, replacements and boosts may be contra-indicated for men with prostate cancer due to possible increased risk of recurrence. One recent study demonstrates the lack of benefits using testosterone replacement for specific parameters (*JAMA*, Vol. 2.99, No. 1, Jan. 2, 2008, pp. 39-52).

These various treatments enable many men with erectile dysfunction to enjoy normal sexual relations. However, one should be realistic about what these methods can and cannot do. Those who suffer from low sexual desire or decreased sensation may not be entirely satisfied with the results that these treatments provide.

Beyond the various treatments for erectile dysfunction, certain changes can be made to counteract other factors that may be contributing to the sexual impairment. Medications that contribute to an erectile problem or a loss of sexual desire can often be exchanged for others that do not have these side effects. Other complications, such as pain or fatigue, may also be contributing factors. Treating these conditions may help. Lifestyle changes, such as improved diet, exercise, quitting smoking, and reduced consumption of alcohol, can also lead to improved sexual performance. When psychological or emotional issues are involved, counseling may serve to decrease performance anxiety and overcome mental blocks to satisfying sex.

CHAPTER ELEVEN

DIETandNUTRITION GUIDELINES

Diet and Prostate Cancer

There is a growing body of evidence that indicates there is a close connection between diet and prostate cancer, as well as other forms of cancer. Other than genetic make-up, no factor has greater influence on a man's likelihood of developing prostate cancer in later life than his diet. We know there is a link between diets high in saturated and total fat and an *increased* risk of prostate cancer. On the other hand, we also know there is a *decreased* risk of prostate cancer with men whose diets are high in fiber, phytoestrogen ("phyto" is Greek for plant), lycopenes (another phyto chemical) and other nutrients.

Recent studies also indicate that dietary habits may improve the prognosis of men already diagnosed with prostate cancer, regardless of stage. It's never too late to change unhealthy eating habits, and it makes good sense for prostate cancer patients to improve their chances for recovery by adopting a healthier diet. If you are undergoing treatment for the disease, your first priority should be to maintain your strength and overall health. In this regard, diet will play an important role before, during and after the treatment process

General Dietary Guidelines

There is no definitive diet for preventing or treating prostate cancer. Specific changes in diet depend on the individual patient. At our institution, we advise patients to consult with a physician or qualified nutritionist for help in developing an individualized diet plan. It should be noted that there is no evidence that diet alone can cure prostate cancer, and therefore, *no one should attempt to use diet or nutritional supplements as substitutes for medical treatment.* However, in general, there are a number of steps that men with prostate cancer can and should take to enhance their prospects for overcoming the disease.

Eat A Low-Fat Diet

Many studies have implicated excessive fat consumption with the development of cancer. The average American man gets approximately 35% or more of his total calories from fat in his diet. The American Cancer Society recommends reducing total fat intake to no more than 30% of total calories for all men and women, including cancer patients. Limiting dietary fat in this way may be especially important in retarding the development of prostate cancer.

A number of studies have demonstrated the link between prostate cancer and a high-fat diet. We know that the incidence of prostate cancer is highest in countries where high-fat diets are prevalent. Prostate cancer is considerably less common among Asian men than men in the U.S., yet the rate of incidence for Asian-Americans who have adopted a typical American diet closely approaches that of other Americans. Studies also show a connection between fat in the diet and mortality rates from prostate cancer. A study from the Harvard School of Public Health found that men with prostate cancer who ate high-fat diets had a 79% greater chance of developing advanced disease. This risk increased significantly when the fat came from red meat.

Given what we know, the most effective way to reduce your risk is to cut down on animal fat in your diet. Favor lean meat and don't eat red meat more than once a week. Instead, you might eat white fish and skinless poultry. Limit your consumption of dairy products. Avoid saturated fats and heavy oils, such as butter, margarine, shortening and corn oil. Instead, polyunsaturated oils, such as olive or safflower oils, should be used in cooking. In addition, avoid heavily processed foods, fast foods and snack foods, all of which are usually high in fat.

The percentage of body fat, not just fats consumed in foods, is also a factor contributing to the growth of prostate cancer. According to the

American Cancer Society, overweight people have roughly twice the cancer mortality rate of people who aren't overweight. Obesity also complicates surgery for prostate cancer, may contribute to symptoms of the disease, and increases the likelihood of heart disease and other health problems. All in all, men with prostate cancer who are significantly overweight would do well to reduce their level of body fat. For patients with an obesity problem, the best course may be a physician-assisted weight loss program, which may also utilize the American Dietetic Soup Diet, Weight Watchers, or similar programs.

If you have prostate cancer and you are one of the millions of Americans who are currently on one of the popular low-carb diets (i.e. the Atkins diet, South Beach diet, the Zone diet), you should consider modifying the plan with your doctor to conform to American Cancer Society recommendations for patients with prostate cancer. The ACS guidelines are similar to those of the American Heart Association and the American Dietetic Association. There is general agreement among nutritionists that a healthy diet involves reducing fat intake and placing more emphasis on fruits and vegetables. The ACS suggests 5 or more servings of fruits and vegetables each day. Grain products, bread, cereals, rice, pasta, and beans are also recommended.

Reduce Cholesterol To Healthy Levels

The media often characterizes cholesterol as a potentially deadly substance, but in reality most cholesterol is manufactured by the body itself for the building of cellular membranes and the formation of vital hormones. The dangers associated with cholesterol occur when supply exceeds demand. Excess cholesterol has been strongly linked to heart attacks and strokes, and may contribute to erectile problems in some men. Although the evidence is so far inconclusive, some researchers suspect high cholesterol may also play a role in prostate cancer.

An overall cholesterol level that exceeds 240 milligrams per deciliter (mg/dl) may signal a problem. But the component elements of blood cholesterol are also relevant. Cholesterol comes in two forms: low-density lipoproteins (LDLs) and high-density lipoproteins (HDLs). Research shows that low levels of high-density lipoproteins may pose as great a health risk as high total cholesterol levels. It appears that higher than average levels of HDL cholesterol can reduce the odds of future health problems. In general, it is wise for men with prostate cancer to reduce their cholesterol levels to around 180 to 200 mg/dl, while maintaining HDL levels at about 45 mg/dl or higher.

Common sense might suggest that the best way to reduce your cholesterol level would be to eat foods low in cholesterol. But dietary cholesterol actually has little impact on blood cholesterol. However, there is a close correlation between dietary fat and the level of serum (blood) cholesterol. Once again, saturated fats are the major offender. Reducing fat intake is the most effective means to lower cholesterol through diet. Substitution of monounsaturated fats for saturated fats will help to lower LDL levels while maintaining the level of HDL's in your bloodstream.

Other dietary changes also have an impact on cholesterol levels. There is evidence that added fiber in the diet can significantly lower cholesterol. Patients are well advised to limit dietary cholesterol from meat and dairy sources to 300 mg/day or less. This is about as much cholesterol as found in 12 ounces of ground beef, 6 ounces of steamed shrimp, or 1 ½ eggs.

Another important factor in managing cholesterol is exercise, which can boost HDL levels by as much as 10% to 20%. In contrast, smoking can significantly reduce HDL levels. When all else fails, certain drugs can effectively treat high cholesterol. Your physician will be able to advise you on whether drug treatment would be appropriate in your case. Also note that all of these diet and lifestyle changes may be enhanced by incorporating relaxation techniques in your daily life.

Maintain A Varied Diet

Most dietary experts recommend a varied diet of nutritious foods. This used to mean that a daily diet should include portions from the four basic food groups: meat, dairy, grains, and fruits and vegetables. The four food groups have since been supplanted by the food pyramid in the U.S. Department of Agriculture's updated dietary guidelines. Breads, cereals, pasta and grains serve as the foundation—three to six servings each day, including several whole grain products. Five to ten servings of fruits and vegetables each day are recommended. Meat, poultry, fish, and other protein sources should be limited to two servings each day. Recommended daily consumption of dairy sources is likewise two servings per day in a healthy diet.

The guidelines are based on research that shows the foundation of a healthy diet to be whole grains, fruits and vegetables. On the other hand, the role of the meat and dairy groups, once seen as staples of a nutritious diet, are significantly diminished. Current USDA recommendations suggest a diet high in fiber, low in fat, and rich in complex carbohydrates. The USDA also strongly advises limiting the consumption of fats, sweets, and alcoholic beverages.

Those contemplating or currently practicing vegetarianism should not interpret the reduced significance of meat and dairy in the new dietary recommendations as sufficient reason for eliminating these food groups entirely. Without proper care, a vegetarian diet may supply inadequate levels of essential amino acids, and could lead to nutritional deficiencies, such as a deficiency of zinc, a mineral central to prostate function. However, with proper planning, a varied vegetarian diet can supply all the essential nutrients.

This underscores the importance of practicing variety within food groups as well. A diet in which vegetable content is supplied only by corn and potatoes will be deficient in many essential nutrients. The relatively recent discovery of phytochemicals, naturally produced chemicals in plants that possess an apparent ability to block carcinogenic processes, indicates that the well-established vitamins and minerals are not the only compounds found in plants that provide health benefits. Frequent rotation of foods, especially whole foods, is one way to ensure a varied, nutritious diet.

Eat Cancer-Fighting Foods

While a healthy diet ought to provide all the nutrients needed by the body, research indicates that certain vitamins, minerals, and chemicals found in foods are particularly useful in combating cancer. These natural substances use a number of mechanisms to protect the body from cancer formation and proliferation. The following may be of use in the fight against prostate cancer:

Vitamin D

Some epidemiological studies, which track broad patterns of diet and disease in the population, suggest that vitamin D may help prevent prostate cancer. In fact, several studies indicate that exposure to sunlight can significantly reduce the risk of prostate cancer, possibly due to the skin's conversion of sunlight into vitamin D. Besides sunlight, the best sources for this vitamin are sardines, fortified milk, and egg yolks.

Antioxidants

This group of nutrients include vitamins A, C, E, selenium and beta-carotene. According to current theory, antioxidants work to block the formation in the body of dangerous forms of oxygen known as free radicals. These free radicals are believed to damage cell membranes, impairing the cell's ability to perform essential tasks, such as control of metabolism, regeneration of internal damage, and elimination of bacteria, viruses and toxins. If this theory is correct, antioxidants may help to short circuit the processes that lead to cancer. Studies thus far have been inconclusive, but including foods in your diet that are rich in antioxidants may be beneficial.

Resveratrol is a unique antioxident that has been shown to act against prostate cancer at all stages and has inspired a great deal of research. A polyphenol found in grapes and other plants, resveratrol is considered a promising agent in the fight against prostate cancer by researchers at MD Anderson Cancer Center and other institutions. Resveratrol works through various anticancer mechanisms and selectively targets cancer cells. It reportedly modulates hormones and has mechanisms that can kill or stop cancer cells from multiplying. One formulation of resveratrol has recently been marketed as Longevinex®.

Overcooking food can eliminate these important nutrients, and because many vitamins are water-soluble, they can be lost through boiling. Therefore, it is best to eat fruits and vegetables raw or steamed. Those patients concerned that their diet is not supplying sufficient quantities of these important nutrients can supplement their diet with a multivitamin. Further supplementation should be undertaken only under a doctor's supervision. In addition, as previously noted, patients undergoing radiation therapy should avoid excessive antioxidants while being treated, as these may have an opposing action to radiation. For more information on specific antioxidants, see Nutritional Supplements below.

Phytochemicals

These substances are naturally occurring chemicals found in plants, apparently serving to protect them from the harmful effects of sunlight. Medical research has shown that phytochemicals also serve as cancer-fighting agents in the human body. A myriad of these biochemicals exist in the fruits and vegetables that we eat—it's been estimated that there are 10,000 in tomatoes alone! Although they have yet to draw the media interest generated by the antioxidants, phytochemicals have caught the attention of private and public institutions in the health industry. The National Cancer Institute has launched a multimillion-dollar project to isolate and study them.

There is some evidence indicating the microscopic activities of these chemicals may slow or reverse the mechanisms that lead to the growth of malignant tumors. Para-coumaric acid and chlorogenic acid, found in tomatoes as well as several other fruits and vegetables, block the formation of carcinogenic compounds called nitrosomes. A phytochemical in turnips eliminates enzymes that cause cellular mutations. Sulforaphane, one of many phytochemicals found in broccoli, has been shown to retard the development of breast tumors in mice.

According to researchers, phytochemicals work by synthesizing enzymes that attach to carcinogenic molecules, dragging them out of the cells before any damage can be done. Citrus fruits, berries, and a number of vegetables contain flavanoids, phytochemicals that prevent cancer-causing hormones from fastening onto cells. These chemicals might be especially advantageous to prostate cancer patients, since most cases of prostate cancer are hormone-dependent.

Another significant finding for men with prostate cancer is a chemical in soybeans called *genistein,* discovered by German researchers. Genistein acts to prevent the formation of capillaries around a malignant tumor, essentially cutting off the tumor's supply lines to impede or halt its growth. This finding has prompted some researchers to suggest that one cause for the high risk of prostate cancer among Asian men who emigrate to the U.S. may be due to the adoption of a soy-poor American diet.

Although synthetic versions of sulforaphane have been created in the laboratory, in all likelihood it will be many years before phytochemicals will be available in a pill. Until then, make sure you eat plenty of whole fruits and vegetables. Fortunately, most phytochemicals appear to hold up through a variety of cooking processes.

Zinc

The prostate gland contains higher concentrations of zinc than any other part of the body. The exact relationship between zinc and the prostate is unknown, but there is some evidence suggesting that a zinc deficiency may precede the development of prostate problems, including prostate cancer. For this reason, eating foods containing zinc may be beneficial. Foods rich in zinc include pumpkin seeds, oysters and other seafood, nuts, wheat bran and wheat germ, milk, eggs, onions, poultry, gelatin, beans, peas, lentils, and beef liver. Overcooking will deplete the natural zinc content of most foods.

Zinc supplements are sometimes prescribed to treat the symptoms of prostate enlargement and prostatitis, and should only be taken under the supervision of a physician. It should also be noted that there is not yet any solid evidence that zinc supplements are effective in treating prostate cancer.

Nutritional Supplements

Vitamins are natural substances that have been scientifically established to be essential for physical health. A deficiency in any of the essential vitamins may result in serious health problems, such as scurvy or rickets (due to deficiencies of vitamins C and D respectively). The development of natural and synthetic vitamin supplements was aimed at the prevention of such deficiencies. Now most deficiencies can be prevented or corrected through the use of nutritional supplements. Taking vitamin or mineral supplements may affect your prostate cancer risk, but this is not yet clear.

The therapeutic value of vitamin and mineral supplements such as antioxidants—vitamins A, C, E, beta-carotene and selenium—is still the subject of debate. When it comes to the health benefits of nutritional supplements in excess of the recommended daily allowances (RDAs), the opinions of physicians and other health professionals vary to some degree. Many conventional physicians question the value of using vitamin megadoses (recommending higher doses than the RDA) as a form of therapy, arguing that megadosing is an expensive and potentially hazardous health fad, driven primarily by profit.

Proponents of the medicinal use of vitamin and mineral megadosing argue that even though scientific proof is inconclusive, the public should not be denied information on potentially beneficial alternatives. No doubt the debate will continue. There are a number of specific antioxidants that may be beneficial for men with prostate cancer, and these are discussed below.

Vitamin A (retinol) and Beta-carotene

In its active form, vitamin A is found only in animal products such as whole milk, eggs, and meat, especially liver. Because many of these foods should be eaten in moderation, it is probably better to rely on the vitamin A precursor, beta-carotene, for this valuable nutrient. Found in a wide range of fruits and vegetables, beta-carotene is essentially two vitamin A molecules linked together. The liver acts to convert beta-carotene into active vitamin A.

Both animal studies and human trials have demonstrated a connection between low levels of these nutrients in the diet and increased risk of a variety of cancers. However, some studies have suggested that vitamin A supplements may actually *increase* the risk of prostate cancer by lowering the level of zinc in the prostate. The evidence to date points to beta-carotene as a better antioxidant and more effective anticancer agent.

When taken at high doses for a prolonged period, vitamin A can cause harmful, even fatal, liver damage. Dietary supplementation with beta-carotene is a much safer approach. Excessive dosages (megadosing) of beta-carotene may increase the risk of lung cancer. Excessive dosing of beta-carotene may cause a yellowing of the skin (carotenosis), but this condition appears to be harmless.

Vitamin C (ascorbic acid)

Nobel Laureate Dr. Linus Pauling, who popularized the use of vitamin C as a remedy for the common cold, also advocated the use of vitamin C supplements for the prevention and treatment of cancer. Vitamin C is not only a powerful antioxidant, but plays an important role in the immune system. During the 1970s, Pauling published several studies that showed high doses of supplemental vitamin C increased survival time for terminal cancer patients. However, at least three randomized trials by the National Cancer Institute failed to confirm Dr. Pauling's findings, and subsequent studies have been inconclusive.

Orange juice, as well as tomatoes, broccoli, Brussels sprouts, cabbage, green peppers, and spinach, are good sources of vitamin C. The RDA for vitamin C is 60 milligrams, but the vitamin is generally considered non-toxic at much higher dosages. The most common side effect of excessive vitamin C is diarrhea. Rare complications have been known to result as a consequence of megadosing. Also, the body becomes conditioned to higher intake of vitamin C, and abrupt cessation of a high dosage could result in a dangerous drop of vitamin C in the blood. Dosages far in excess of nutritional needs should only be taken in consultation with a physician.

Vitamin E

This antioxidant vitamin has been the subject of much attention. Foods rich in vitamin E include green leafy vegetables, whole grains, and veg-etable oils. Like vitamin A, vitamin E is a fat-soluble vitamin that collects in the body. Researchers caution that the safety of vitamin E megadoses taken over an extended period has not yet been established.

Some studies suggest that taking 50 milligrams (or 400 International Units) of vitamin E daily can lower risk for prostate cancer. Although other studies found vitamin E to be of no benefit, reasonable doses of this vita-min have no significant side effects and are not expensive. Vitamin E works synergistically with selenium in the body, and taking them in conjunction may enhance their beneficial properties.

Selenium

Found in meat, seafood and whole grains, selenium is an essential trace mineral needed by the body for pancreatic function and to maintain tissue elasticity. Selenium is also a broad-spectrum antioxidant. Studies have shown that selenium and vitamin E work together to aid in the production of antibodies. Animal studies have found selenium retards tumor formation. Other studies suggest that ending selenium supplementation in animals can result in an increase in tumor development. Therefore, those who advocate taking selenium to prevent cancer also caution against sudden cessation of supplementation.

As with vitamins A, C, and E, several studies have found that individuals with low serum selenium levels had a significantly higher risk of developing cancer. A large-scale NCI study—the Selenium and Vitamin E Cancer Prevention Trial (SELECT)—was halted in 2008 when it found no benefits after more than five years. However, this finding contradicts earlier data, including population based studies.

Some patients have difficulty absorbing selenium when taken as oral supplements. Caution should be practiced in taking large doses of selenium, since the mineral can be quite toxic. Bad breath is one harmless side effect of selenium megadoses, but more severe symptoms can result as a consequence of selenium toxicity. These include nausea and weakness. There may also be discoloration of the fingernails. Close medical supervision and testing of blood selenium levels is necessary to prevent toxicity in those taking large doses of selenium.

Additional Suggestions

The patient is the one who must finally decide whether or not to take nutritional supplements. The safest route—and one recommended by the FDA—is to get your antioxidants in the foods you eat every day. Nevertheless, you may wish to take more aggressive action. If a blood test indicates that you have low levels of key nutrients in your bloodstream, you may be more likely to benefit from supplements. But keep in mind that megadosages can be hazardous, and some supplements may interact with various medications or pose a health risk for men with medical conditions other than prostate cancer. Always seek the advice of a physician before beginning any vitamin regimen.

Although much has been made of studies indicating the promise of antioxidants as cancer-fighting agents, nutritional supplements are no substitute for a proper diet and healthy lifestyle. Don't make them a substitute for practicing healthy habits in your life.

In addition, it should be noted again that supplements may help to prevent prostate cancer, but after cancer is diagnosed, they will not bring about a cure. All prostate cancer patients require appropriate medical treatment to be cured or to minimize progression of the disease.

Summary of Diet and Nutrition Guidelines

At the Dattoli Cancer Center, patients who are being treated for prostate cancer are routinely advised as follows, with appropriate updates as new studies continually improve our current knowledge:

In general, eat healthy with a higher protein, lower fat diet

Adopt a mainly vegan diet consisting of fruits and vegetables (5 servings a day), and legumes. Minimize or eliminate red meat entirely. Chicken and fish are best if broiled or baked. Fish should be lean (and oily) like Salmon, Tuna, Anchovies, Sardines, Mackerel (which also contains Omega-3 acids). Make sure to remove skin from chicken before cooking. Avoid all fried foods.

Increase fiber intake

Eat at least 3 servings of whole grains daily. Limit white starches and increase whole grains such as whole wheat breads and crackers, wheat pasta, brown or wild rice, whole grain cereals, wheat pita bread, brown rice cakes, barley, oats, millet, quinoa, and spelt.

Increase Phytoestrogen intake

Concentrate on soybeans and soy products, legumes (beans), bean sprouts, sunflower seeds, rye, wheat and all berries. Also note that members of the cabbage family (broccoli, cauliflower, onions, radishes, horseradish) have been shown to be beneficial for cancer patients.

Increase Lycopene intake

Increase consumption of tomato-based foods, such as tomato sauce, pizza, and tomatoes. While at least one recent study (2007) questions the value of lycopene and multivitamins specifically with regard to prostate cancer, Dr. Dattoli questions the methodology employed by those researchers. Previous studies suggesting the benefits of lycopene and multivitamins appear to be more reliable.

Eat more cold water fish for their high omega 3 polyunsaturated fat content

Choose wild salmon, haddock, halibut, cod, pink tuna, herring, sardines, and arctic char. You might also include flounder, shellfish, grouper or snapper, although they do not contain high levels of omega 3 fats. Avoid King mackerel, shark, and albacore tuna due to their high mercury contents.

Avoid red meat and pork

These have high levels of saturated fats and arachidonic acid which is believed to promote prostate cancer growth. If you must have beef, then choose grass-fed beef, and then only once a week. Pork is the worst meat you can eat due to what pigs are fed. Choose white meat chicken and turkey, egg whites and Egg Beaters. Also include plant protein sources such as beans, lentils, soy, nuts, and nut butters.

Avoid fats and oils

Use less butter, margarine, oil and high-fat salad dressings. Use olive oil instead. Consume less cheese, or use fat-free or low-fat cheeses. Eat fewer desserts, or choose low-fat or fat-free desserts.

Avoid, or at least limit, dairy foods such as milk, cheese, yogurt, and ice cream

Instead, use non-fat dairy products (skim milk, non-fat cheese and ice cream). Or better yet, use the soy alternatives. Try soy in the form of tofu, tempeh, miso, soy milk, yogurt, ice cream, soy cheeses, ground round, meatballs, and burgers. Their isoflavone content may be beneficial for cancer prevention.

Avoid foods high in sugar content

They create blood sugar swings that affect energy levels. Also, high sugar foods are generally low in nutrients. Sugar depletes the immune system by slowing the action of your white blood cells. Eat fewer desserts, or choose low-fat or fat-free desserts.

Drink 8–10 cups of water daily

Water helps to transport toxins out of the body. You can count decaffeinated beverages toward your water intake, such as flavored club soda, green and black teas, and herbal teas.

Eliminate caffeinated beverages

Caffeine is an irritant and dehydrates cells. Caffeine drinks include coffee, regular tea, and soda. Red wine in moderation (4 ounces daily) may be beneficial. Likewise, dark chocolate may be beneficial, also in moderation.

Exercise on a regular basis

Without overdoing it, try to exercise at least 30 minutes on most days of the week. Exercise activities might include walking, jogging, swimming, exercise equipment, light weights, etc. At the same time that you address diet and fitness, find a form of stress management that works for you. Some type of meditation or yoga for 20 minutes once or twice daily may be helpful for stress relief.

Take immune-boosting and detoxifying supplements as approved by your physician.

Incorporate as many of the following in your daily diet as possible:

- ➤ **Soy products**—soy milk or powder, or genistein. These inhibit prostate cancer growth and its capacity to spread (metastasize). Or you might take soy isoflavone tablets, 100-130 mg—one table twice daily.

- ➤ **Green Tea**—2-3 cups per day (or capsules). Green tea boosts the immune system and induces prostate cancer programmed cell death (apoptosis)

- ➤ **Pomegranate juice**—8 oz. daily. Pomegranate juice offers an antioxidant that delays rise in PSA (doubling time indicating tumor growth), as well as helping promote penile blood flow to reduce erectile dysfunction.

- ➤ **Red grapes or concentrate** (Concord grape juice). Consume daily to protect against bladder dysfunction and potentially improve urinary symptoms.

- ➤ **Lycopenes**—tomato food sources (juice, sauces, etc.) are preferred but lycopenes can also be taken in pill form (30mg-45mg daily).

- **Vitamin C**–500 mg.
- **Vitamin D**–4000-5000 i.u. daily, in cholecalciferol form.
- **Vitamin E**–50-200 i.u. (a combination of gamma and alpha tocopherol is preferred). Vitamin E has been shown to reduce prostate cancer related deaths (upwards of 40%).
- **Calcium Citrate**–400 mg at dinner, 400mg at bedtime. Contributes to bone health.
- **Fish Oil Omega 3** (with or without rosemary)–2000 mg. two times daily. Fish oil Omega 3 inhibits inflammatory response in the body, thereby inhibiting prostate cancer cellular growth and decreasing the potential for cancer to metastasize.
- **Melatonin**–3 to 6 mg. taken nightly if you are having trouble sleeping. Melatonin is an antioxidant that potentially increases longer survival from cancer and potentially reduces side effects of treatment related to stress, gastrointestinal and renal (kidney) factors.
- **Selenium**–200 mcg. Selenium has been shown to decrease prostate cancer related deaths.
- **Zinc**–50-100 mg. Zinc protects normal cells and increases prostate cancer cell death.
- **Indole-3-Carbinol**–200–400 mg. daily. Indole-3-Carbinol is an anti-cancer compound found in cruciferous vegetables that decreases the risk of developing cancer.
- **Modified Citrus Pectin**–800 mg. three times daily taken with meals.
- **Quercetin**–as per instructions (found in health food stores) for general prostate health. You may also use a combination product with Chrysin and Saw Palmetto called Sports One Chrysin XS. Quercetin may reduce the expression of p53, thereby inhibiting angiogenesis and the growth of prostate cancer.

➤ **Glutamine**—2 grams with each meal and at bedtime. Glutamine contributes to muscle strength for patients undergoing hormonal therapy.

➤ **Glucosamine**—1500mg (NOT to be combined with chondroitin). Glucosamine helps with joint/bone strength for patients undergoing hormonal therapy. Chondroitin can potentially cause increased recurrence rates and progression of cancer.

➤ **Beta-Sitosterol**—100-200 mg. daily. This is the most active constituent of pygeum, and it has anti-inflammatory effects to prostate tissue.

➤ **Cernitin**—2-4 tablets daily for general prostate health. Cernitin has anti-inflammatory properties and is used for chronic prostatitis symptoms.

There are a number of prostate antioxidant formulas found in most pharmacies and health food stores, and these may contain the majority of these supplements. They may be easier to take than separate doses of each item above. If you elect to take one of these preparations, make sure it contains folic acid.

More Diet Guidelines

Another comprehensive source on diet guidelines for prostate cancer patients can be found on-line in the publication, *Eating Your Way to Better Health: The Prostate Forum Nutrition Guide,* compiled by Charles E. Myers, Jr., M.D., et al. For more information, visit the Prostate Forum website at:

www.prostateforum.com/nutrition.htm

The article, "Nutrition for Healing After Prostate Cancer," by Pamela Mathis, M.Ed., R.D., L.D. also offers comprehensive nutritional guidelines for patients and is available upon request from the Dattoli Cancer Center (see *Appendix A: Where To Get Help*).

WHERE TO GET HELP

Your Physician

A trusted physician who is familiar with your case should be your most important source of information and advice. For those who desire additional information, there are a number of organizations devoted to helping prostate cancer patients and their families. These agencies provide information and counseling, and in some cases, they may provide financial aid and/or transportation to a medical facility for treatment.

Organizations and Businesses

The following is a list of national organizations and medical centers that provide information and services for prostate cancer patients. For information on local support groups, contact the social service office of a local hospital, or write or call one of the national cancer information services listed below.

American Cancer Society (ACS)

1599 Clifton Road, N.E. Atlanta, GA 30329
(800) ACS-2345
http://www.cancer.org

Man To Man Prostate Cancer Support Groups

The American Cancer Society is involved in education and research, and offers counseling and other patient services. The Society consists of more than 3000 local chapters across the United States, and has adopted the Man to Man prostate cancer support group program on a national basis.

American Foundation of Urologic Disease
300 West Pratt Street, Suite 401, Baltimore, MD 21201-2463
(800) 242-2383
http://www.afud.org

Amersham Healthcare
Medi-Physics, Inc., 101 Carnegie Center, Princeton, NJ 08540
(800) 654-0118
http://www.amershamhealth-us.com

Medi-Physics is the manufacturer of the radioactive iodine seeds used in brachytherapy for the treatment of early stage prostate cancer. The company readily supplies information to those wanting to know more about seed implantation and Medi-Physics products. Medi-Physics also makes available listings of doctors who perform the seed implantation procedure.

Cancer Information Service (CIS)
National Cancer Institute (NCI) Building 31, Room 10A24 9000
Rockville Pike Bethesda, MD 20892
(800) 4-CANCER
http://cis.nci.nih.gov/

A governmental service that provides information by telephone and via Web site to cancer patients, the public, and health care professionals. Trained staff members can provide information on current treatments, cancer prevention, and the nearest Comprehensive Cancer Center. The National Cancer Institute also supplies a wide variety of written materials to answer questions about cancer. The PDQ, or Physician Data Query, is a computer information system that provides doctors and patients with the latest information on clinical trials and their results. The Cancer Information Service will provide a copy of the PDQ to anyone who requests it.

Dattoli Cancer Center
2803 Fruitville Road, Sarasota, FL 34237
(877) 328-8654 toll free
http://www.dattoli.com

The Dattoli Cancer Center & Brachytherapy Research Institute specializes in combined treatment modalities and often pairs brachytherapy with

4-Dimensional Image Guided-Intensity Modulated Radiation Therapy (4D IG-IMRT). The authors of this book are affiliated with this facility.

Dattoli Cancer Foundation

2803 Fruitville Road, Sarasota, FL 34237

(800) 915-1001

http://www.dattolifoundation.com

http://www.prostatetreatment.org

The nonprofit arm of the Dattoli Cancer Center, whose mission is to raise awareness of prostate cancer, provide current and accurate information on diagnosis and treatment, and support the research of the Dattoli Cancer Center physicians. Numerous books and booklets are available, as well as a speaker's bureau.

Foundation for Cancer Research and Education

P.O. Box 746, Earlysville, VA 22936

(800) 305-2432

http://www.cancer-foundation.org

Prostate Cancer prevention and treatment information researched by Dr. Charles "Snuffy" Myers, Jr. Publishes "Prostate Forum" newsletter, and several respected books, including *Eating Your Way to Better Health: The Prostate Forum Nutrition Guide.*

Impotence Institute of America

8201 Corporate Drive, Suite 320, Landover, MD 20715

(800) 669-1603

http://www.impotenceworld.org

Impotence Anonymous

A division of the Impotence World Assocation, the Impotence Institute of America (IIA) is a nonprofit organization dedicated to helping men with impotence problems and their partners. The Institute provides information and physician referrals, and is sponsor of Impotence Anonymous, a support group with chapters in most major metropolitan centers.

Man To Man

c/o American Cancer Society
1599 Clifton Road, N.E. Atlanta, GA 30329
(800) ACS-2345
http://www.cancer.org/docroot/SHR/content/SHR_2.1_x_Man_to_Man.
asp?sitearea=SHR

Man To Man is a national support group officially sponsored by the American Cancer Society to provide information and support to men with prostate cancer and their families. To find out more about Man To Man, contact the American Cancer Society at the address and phone number listed above.

National Association for Continence

P.O. Box 8306, Spartansburg, SC 29305 (864) 579-7900
http://www.nafc.org

Formerly called Help for Incontinent People (HIP), the National Assocation for Continence is a nonprofit organization that provides information and services to those suffering from incontinence problems.

Patient Advocates for Advanced Cancer Treatments (PAACT)

1143 Parmelee NW, Grand Rapids, MI 49504
(616) 453-1477
http://www.paactusa.org

A nonprofit organization for both patients and physicians that promotes an understanding of prostate cancer, its diagnosis and therapeutic treatment. PAACT has a database on thousands of patients with prostate cancer, and readily provides information concerning treatment options by telephone and e-mail to those diagnosed with prostate cancer.

Prostate Cancer Research Institute (PCRI)

5777 W. Century Blvd., Suite 885, Los Angeles, CA 90045
Helpline: 310-743-2110
http://www.prostate-cancer.org

The Prostate Cancer Research Institute is a non-profit organization that offers information to patients and physicians.

Theragenics Corporation

5325 Oakbrook Parkway Norcross, GA 30093

(800) 458-4372

http://www.theragenics.com

Theragenics is the largest manufacturer of the radioactive palladium seeds used in brachytherapy for the treatment of prostate cancer. The company supplies information to those interested in knowing more about the seed implantation procedure and Theragenics' products. Theragenics will also refer interested patients to a physician who offers the seed implantation treatment in their general area.

US TOO Support Groups

US TOO, Inc. 5003 Fairview Avenue, Downers Grove, IL 60515

(630) 795-1002

PCa Support Hotline: (800) 80-US-TOO

http://www.ustoo.com/

The mission of US TOO!™, is to provide counseling, fellowship, and support to cancer patients and their families. Contact the national headquarters of US TOO!™ at the address and number above to find out where your nearest US TOO!™ chapter is located.

Varian Medical Systems, Inc.

1678 S. Pioneer Road, Salt Lake City UT 84104

(800) 432-4422

http://www.varian.com/com

Varian specializes in manufacturing integrated cancer therapy systems, including Intensity Modulated Radiation Therapy and brachytherapy.

Veterans Affairs (VA) Hospitals and Support Services

The Department of Veterans Affairs (VA) supports veterans seeking the benefits and services earned through military service. For Vietnam veterans, benefits may include disability compensation, health care services, tax breaks, and more. For more information about these programs, call the VA's toll-free Agent Orange Helpline at 1-800-749-8387, or go to the web site at www.vva.org/benefits/vvgagent.htm. The home page for the Department of Veterans Affairs is located at http://www.va.gov/. For questions about VA healthcare benefits, call toll free 1-877-222-8387.

Internet Resources

The following is a list of specialized Web sites devoted to prostate cancer information and support:

Prostate Pointers
http://www.prostatepointers.org

Prostate Cancer Foundation is the renamed Michael Milken CaP Cure
http://www.prostatecancerfoundation.org/

National Prostate Cancer Coalition:
http://www.pcacoalition.org/

National Cancer Institute's Prostate Cancer Home Page:
http://www.cancer.gov/cancerinfo/types/prostate

The Hypertext Guide to Prostate Cancer:
http://www.hypertext.org

Florida Cancer Education Network:
http://www.florida-prostate-cancer.org/

Prostate Cancer InfoLink Archive:
http://www.phoenix5.org/Infolink/index.html

PPML website:
http://listserv.acor.org/diseases/prostate

PPML archives:
http://listserv.acor.org/archives/prostate.html

MultiGraph: your medical history in graphic form, free from PC-REF:
Contact John Fistere at JFistere@cox.net
http://members.cox.net/jfistere/MultiGraphIntro.htm

WellnessWeb Prostate Cancer Center:
http://www.wellnessweb.com/PROSTATE/prostate.htm

Center for Prostate Disease Research:
http://www.cpdr.org/

Patients Helping Patients:
http://www.prostate-help.org/

Malecare: lecture transcripts, English and Spanish New York City support groups:
http://www.malecare.com

Canadian Prostate Cancer Network:
http://www.cpcn.org/

Brotherhood of the Balloon—Proton Therapy Info and Support:
http://www.protonbob.com/homepage.asp

PSA Rising Magazine:
http://www.psa-rising.com

Prostate Cancer Action Network:
http://www.prostatepointers.org/pcan/

Pubmed search—a comprehensive listing of research studies and published papers:
http://www.ncbi.nlm.nih.gov/entrez/query.fcgi

GLOSSARY OF MEDICAL TERMS

3D-CRT (3-Dimensional Conformal Radiation Therapy): See Conformal Radiotherapy.

5-alpha reductase (5-AR): an enzyme that converts testosterone to dihydrotestosterone (DHT).

Adenocarcinoma: A cancer originating in glandular tissue. Prostate cancer is classified as adenocarcinoma of the prostate.

Adjuvant: An additional treatment used to increase the effectiveness of the primary therapy. Radiation therapy and hormonal therapy are often used as adjuvant treatments following a radical prostatectomy. Compare Neoadjuvant.

Agonist: A chemical substance that combines with a receptor on a cell and initiates an activity or reaction. See LHRH analogs.

Algorithm: A step-by-step procedure for solving a problem or accomplishing some end, especially by a computer.

Analog: A man-made chemical compound that is structurally similar to one produced naturally by the body. See LHRH analogs.

Androgen: A hormone that produces male characteristics. See testosterone.

Androgen ablation therapy: A therapy designed to inhibit the body's production of testosterones.

Androgen-dependent cells: Prostate cancer cells which are nourished by male hormones and therefore are capable of being destroyed by hormone deprivation (also known as androgen-sensitive cells).

Androgen-independent cells: Prostate cancer cells which are not dependent on male hormones and therefore do not respond to hormonal therapy (also known as androgen-insensitive cells).

Androgens: The male hormones, such as testosterone.

Anesthetic: A drug that produces general or local loss of physical sensations, particularly pain. A "spinal" is the injection of a local anesthetic into the area surrounding the spinal cord.

Aneuploid: Having an abnormal number of chromosomes, as revealed by ploidy analysis. Aneuploid prostate cancer cells tend not to respond well to androgen deprivation therapy (ADT).

Angiogenesis: The body's formation of new blood vessels. Some anti-cancer drugs work by blocking angiogenesis, thus preventing blood from reaching and nourishing a tumor.

Antagonist: A chemical substance in the body that acts to reduce the physiological activity of another chemical substance.

Anti-androgens: Drugs such as flutamide that block the activity of androgens produced by the adrenal glands at the cellular receptor sites. Androgens can block or neutralize the effects of testosterone and DHT on prostate cancer cells (by preventing testosterone and DHT from binding to the androgen receptor).

Antibody: A protein produced by the body that counteracts the toxic effects of a foreign substance, organism, or disease within the body.

Antigen: A foreign substance such as a virus or bacterium that causes an immune response or the formation of an antibody.

Antioxidants: Any substances which delay the process of oxidation in the body.

Apoptosis: The normal molecular mechanism which governs the life span of cells so that they die in a very organized way. Cancerous cells are resistant to normal apoptosis.

Benign: A non-cancerous condition. See also Benign Prostatic Hypertrophy.

Benign Prostatic Hypertrophy (BPH): Also called Benign Prostatic Hyperplasia, BPH is a non-cancerous condition of the prostate that results in a growth of tumorous tissue and increase in the size of the prostate.

Biopsy: A procedure involving the removal of tissue from the body of the patient. Removed tissue is typically examined microscopically by a pathologist in order to make a precise diagnosis of the patient's condition.

Bone scan: An imaging technique used to detect bone metastases, which appear as "hot spots" on the film. It is far more sensitive than the conventional x-ray.

BPH: See Benign Prostatic Hypertrophy.

Brachytherapy: A form of radiation therapy in which radioactive seeds are implanted into the prostate to deliver radiation directly to the tumor. Also referred to as seed implantation, or seeding.

Cancer: A cellular malignancy typically forming tumors. Unlike benign tumors, these tend to invade surrounding tissues and spread to distant sites of the body.

Carcinoma: A malignant tumor made up chiefly of epithelial cells, or those cells that form the lining of an organ or cavity. See Adenocarcinoma.

Castrate Range: The level of the body's testosterone after orchiectomy (also referred to as castration). This is the range or level, which is used by physicians as a point of comparison for those drugs, which attempt to decrease the testosterone level.

CAT Scan (or CT Scan): See Computer Tomography.

cGy: Abbreviation for centigray; a unit of radiation equivalent to the older unit called a "rad."

Chemotherapy: The treatment of cancer using chemicals that deter the growth of cancer cells.

Collimator: A device that organizes radiation such that only parallel rays or beams emanate.

Combination Hormonal Therapy (CHT): Also referred to as Combined Hormonal Blockade (CHB), or Combined Androgen Deprivation Therapy (ADT). The preferred term is ADT, often designated with a number referring to the number of agents used (i.e., monotherapy ADT, ADT2, ADT3). This combined therapy can utilize a number of mechanisms, including surgical or medical ADT, anti-androgens, 5-alpha reductase inhibitors, estrogenic compounds, agents that block adrenal androgen production, and agents that decrease the receptivity of the androgen receptor.

Combination Therapy: Refers generally to any combination of treatment modalities used to treat prostate cancer.

Computer Tomography: Computer generated cross-sectional images of a portion of the body. Also called CT or CAT scan.

Conformal Radiotherapy: A radiation treatment conforming precisely to the size and shape of the prostate, with the use of computerized planning and state-of-the-art imaging techniques. 3-Dimensional Conformal Radiation Therapy (3D-CRT) utilizes this sophisticated approach to treatment planning, as does the even more advanced Intensity Modulated Radiation Therapy (IMRT).

Cryosurgery (also referred to as Cryotherapy or Cryoablation): The freezing of tissue with the use of liquid nitrogen or Argon gas probes. When used to treat prostate cancer, the cryoprobes are guided by transrectal ultrasound.

Cytokine: Any of a class of immunoregulatory substances that are secreted by cells of the immune system.

DHT (dihydrotestosterone): The active form of the male hormone, testosterone, produced after testosterone is transformed by an enzyme known as 5-alpha reductase.

Diagnosis: Evaluation of a patient's symptoms and/or test results, with the intent of identifying and verifying the existence of any underlying disease or abnormal condition.

Digital Rectal Examination (DRE): A procedure in which the physician inserts a gloved, lubricated finger into the rectum to examine the prostate gland for signs of cancer.

DNA (Deoxyribonucleic Acid): A complex protein that is the carrier of genetic information that determines the physical development and growth of living organisms.

Doppler Ultrasound Technique: A machine that sends out ultrasonic waves that pick up the velocity of blood flow through the veins and are transmitted as sound to make an image.

Doubling Time: The time it takes for a tumor or cancerous focus to double in size.

Downsizing: The use of hormonal therapy or other forms of intervention to reduce tumor volume prior to primary, curative treatment.

Downstaging: The use of hormonal therapy or other forms of intervention to lower the clinical stage of prostate cancer prior to primary, curative treatment.

Ejaculatory Ducts: The tubular passages through which semen reaches the prostatic urethra during orgasm.

Ejaculation: The release of semen through the penis during orgasm.

Endorectal MRI: Magnetic resonance imaging of the prostate gland using a probe inserted into the rectum.

Enzyme: A chemical substance produced by living cells that causes chemical reactions to take place while not being changed itself.

Erectile Dysfunction (also referred to as ED or impotence): The loss of ability to produce and/or sustain an erection sufficient for intercourse.

Estrogen: A female sex hormone that can be used as a form of therapy to inhibit the production of testosterone in patients diagnosed with prostate. cancer.

Eulexin®: See flutamide.

External Beam Radiation Therapy (EBRT): A form of radiation therapy that utilizes radiation delivered by an external source (machine) and directed at a target area to be radiated. In contrast to EBRT, brachytherapy utilizes radiation sources (seeds) that are internal, implanted in the target tissue. EBRT may use conventional photons, protons, neutrons or electrons.

Extracapsular Extension: Used to describe prostate cancer that has spread outside the prostate gland.

False Negative: An erroneous negative test result. For example, an imaging test that fails to show the presence of a cancer tumor later found by biopsy to be present in the patient is said to have returned a false negative result.

False Positive: A positive test result that mistakenly identifies a state or condition that does not in fact exist.

Fistula: With regard to prostate cancer, an abnormal passage due to injury or disease that connects an abscess or hollow organ to the surface of the body or to another hollow organ. If there is significant damage to the rectal wall proximate to the bladder, a fistula may occur between the bladder and rectum.

Flare Reaction: A testosterone surge caused by the initial use of an LHRH analog, causing a temporary increase of tumor growth and symptoms (known as clinical flare), or an increase in PSA (biochemical flare).

Flutamide: The generic name of Eulexin®, an anti-androgen used in hormonal therapy for the palliative treatment of advanced prostate cancer and for adjuvant and neoadjuvant treatment of earlier stages of prostate cancer.

Foley Catheter: A catheter inserted in the penis and threaded through the urethra to the bladder where it is held in place with a tiny, inflated balloon. It removes urine from the bladder and can be used to irrigate the urethra and prevent blood clots.

Free PSA: PSA that is unattached to any major protein in the blood. Free PSA is associated with benign prostate growth. The percentage of free PSA is derived by dividing the free-PSA level by the total-PSA x 100. Studies have show that men with free PSA % > 25% were at low risk for prostate cancer, while men with PSA % < 10% were at high risk for having prostate cancer.

Frozen Section: A technique in which removed tissue is frozen, cut into thin slices, and stained for microscopic examination. A pathologist can rapidly complete a frozen section analysis, and for this reason, it is commonly used during surgery to quickly provide the surgeon with vital information.

Gland: An aggregation of cells (a structure or organ) that secretes a substance for use or discharge from the body.

Gland Volume: The size in cubic centimeters (cc) or grams of the prostate gland.

Gleason Score: A widely used method for classifying the cellular differentiation of cancerous tissue. The less the cancerous cells appear like normal cells, the more malignant the cancer. Two grades of 1-5, identifying the two most common degrees of differentiation present in the examined tissue sample, are added together to produce the Gleason score. High numbers indicate greater differentiation and more aggressive cancer. The grading system is named after its originator, Donald Gleason, M.D.

Globulin: Any of a number of simple proteins that occur widely in plant and animal tissues.

Gynecomastia: A side effect involving breast enlargement and tenderness, associated with various hormonal therapies that increase the level of estrogens in the body.

HDR brachytherapy: High Dose Rate brachytherapy involves the temporary insertion of radioactive iridium isotopes into the prostate gland using transrectal ultrasound guidance.

Hematuria: Blood in the urine.

Hereditary: Inherited genetically from parents and earlier generations.

Holistic Medicine: Medical care, which considers the patient as a whole, including his or her physical, mental, emotional, spiritual, social and economic needs.

Hormone: A substance produced by one tissue or gland and transported by the bloodstream to another to effect or regulate physiological activity such as metabolism and growth.

Hormonal therapy: Cancer treatment involving the blockage of hormone production by surgical or chemical means. Because prostate cancer is usually dependent on male hormones to grow, hormonal therapy can be an effective means of alleviating symptoms and retarding the development of the disease.

Hormone refractory prostate cancer: Prostate cancer that is androgen independent, and therefore, unresponsive to hormonal therapies.

Hot Flash: A side effect of some forms of hormonal therapy, experienced as a sudden rush of warmth to the face, neck, and upper body.

Imaging: Radiology techniques that are often computer-enhanced and allow the physician to visualize areas inside the body that would not normally be visible.

Impotence: See Erectile Dysfunction.

Incontinence: A loss of urinary control. There are various kinds and degrees of incontinence. Overflow incontinence is a condition in which the bladder retains urine after voiding. As a consequence, the bladder remains full most of the time, resulting in involuntary seepage of urine from the bladder. Stress incontinence is the involuntary discharge of urine when there is increased pressure upon the bladder, as in coughing or straining to lift heavy objects. Total incontinence is the failure of ability to voluntarily exercise control over the sphincters of the bladder neck and urethra, resulting in total loss of retentive ability.

Inflammation: Redness or swelling caused by injury or infection.

Informed Consent: Permission to proceed given by a patient after being fully informed of the purposes and potential consequences of a medical procedure.

Intensity Modulated Radiation Therapy (IMRT): The most recent state-of-the-art, computer-aided technique for delivering higher doses of radiation more accurately than either conventional External Beam Radiation or Conformal Radiation.

Intermittent Androgen Deprivation (IAD): A temporary discontinuation of hormonal therapy that allows for a return to natural testosterone production in order to spare the patient from symptoms associated with androgen deprivation. Also referred to as Intermittent Hormonal Therapy (IHT).

Intravenous Pyelogram (IVP): A test that utilizes the injection of a special dye to check for injury or the spread of cancer to the kidneys and bladder.

Investigational: A drug or procedure allowed by the FDA for use in clinical trials.

Isodose Line: A line or two-dimensional shape that circumscribes an area receiving a radiation dose greater than or equal to a specified amount.

Laparoscopic Lymphadenectomy: The removal of pelvic lymph nodes with a laparoscope via four small incisions in the lower abdomen.

LH (Luteinizing Hormone): A chemical signal originating in the pituitary gland that causes the testes to make testosterone.

LHRH Analogs (or LHRH Agonists): Synthetic compounds that are chemically similar to Luteinizing Hormone Releasing Hormone (LHRH), used to suppress testicular production of testosterone. The most commonly prescribed LHRH analogs are Lupron® and Zoldex®. See also Luteinizing Hormone-Releasing Hormone (LHRH).

LHRH Antagonist: A chemical agent that blocks the LHRH receptor without the testosterone surge associated with LHRH analogs. LHRH antagonists include Abarelix (Plenaxis®).

Linear Accelerator: A high energy x-ray machine generating radiation fields for external beam radiation therapy. These machines are typically mounted with a collimator (or multileaf collimator) in a gantry that rotates vertically around the patient being treated.

Localized Prostate Cancer: Cancer that is confined to the prostate gland, and therefore, considered curable.

Luteinizing Hormone-Releasing Hormone (LHRH): A chemical signal originating in the hypothalamus that causes the pituitary to make LH, which in turn stimulates the testicles to make testosterone.

Lymphadenectomy: The removal and examination of lymph nodes to precisely diagnose and stage cancer. See also Laparascopic Lymphadenectomy.

Lymph Node: A small, bean-shaped mass of tissue located throughout the body along the vessels of the lymphatic system. The lymph nodes filter out bacteria and other toxins, as well as cancer cells.

Magnetic Resonance Imaging (MRI): A painless, non-invasive technique using strong magnetic fields to produce detailed images of internal body structures. An MRI scan usually takes about 45 minutes.

Malignancy: A tumorous growth of cancer cells.

Malignant: Having the invasive and metastatic properties of cancer. Tending to become progressively worse and to result in death.

Margin: See Surgical Margin.

Metalloprotease Inhibitors: Drugs used to suppress the body's production of certain enzymes.

Metastasis: The spread of cancer, by way of the blood stream or lymphatic system, beyond the boundaries of the organ or structure where the cancer originated. Metastases is the plural. Metastatic refers to the characteristics associated with cancer that has spread or a secondary tumor.

Metastatic Work-Up: A group of tests, including bone scans, x-rays, and blood tests, to ascertain whether cancer has metastasized.

Monoclonal Antibody (mAb): An antibody that is directed against one specific protein (antigen).

Morbidity: Unhealthy consequences and complications resulting from treatment.

MRI: See Magnetic Resonance Imaging.

Nadir: The lowest point. Doctors sometimes use this as a verb to describe return of cancer or treatment failure. The PSA nadir refers to a minimum PSA value that should be maintained after treatment if the cancer has been successfully eradicated.

Necrosis: Death of cells or tissues caused by disease or injury.

Neoadjuvant: The use of a different type of therapy before primary, curative treatment. For example, neoadjuvant Androgen Deprivation Therapy is often used prior to radiation therapy or radical surgery, with the intent of improving the effectiveness of the primary treatment by reducing the size of the tumor and/or prostate gland.

Nerve-sparing: A procedure used during radical prostatectomy in which the surgeon attempts to save the nerves (neurovascular bundles) that allow for normal sexual functions.

Neurovascular Bundles: Strands of interwoven nerves and veins that run down the side of the prostate. The bundles contain microscopic nerves that are essential for erection; they also contain arteries and veins. Cutting the nerves in the bundles during surgery, or otherwise harming them in another procedure, usually renders the patient impotent.

Nocturia: Getting up at night to urinate.

Non-invasive: Not involving any incision in the body.

Oncogenes: Genes associated with tumor growth.

Oncology: The branch of medical science dealing with tumors. A medical oncologist is a specialist in the study of cancerous tumors.

Organ-confined Disease (OCD): Prostate cancer that is confined to the prostate capsule, as indicated clinically or pathologically.

Orchiectomy: A simple operation that involves surgical removal of the testicles, which produce most of the body's testosterone.

Osteoporosis: A decrease in bone mass and density causing fragility and porosity.

Overstaging: An assessment of an overly high clinical stage at initial diagnosis.

Palpable: Capable of being felt when examined by touch or manipulation.

PAP: See Prostatic Acid Phosphatase.

Pathologist: A doctor who specializes in the examination of cells and tissues removed from the body.

PBRT: See Proton Beam Radiation Therapy.

Perineum: The area of the body between the anus and scrotum. A perineal procedure uses this area as the point of entry into the body.

Perineural Invasion: Describing cancer, which has spread from the prostate to the nerve bundles.

Periprostatic: Relating to the soft tissues immediately proximate to the prostate gland.

Photon: The quantum of electromagnetic energy, described as having zero mass and no electric charge. X-rays are high energy photons.

Placebo: A sugar pill often taken by participants in a medical study. Patients taking a placebo are compared to patients taking actual medications.

Ploidy Analysis: A pathological analysis to determine the number of sets of chromosomes in a cell.

Proctitis: Inflammation of the rectum.

Prognosis: A forecast of the course of a disease and future prospects of the patient.

Progression: A change in the status of the cancer indicating the condition has progressed and worsened.

Pro-oxidant: A term to describe substances that aid in oxidation.

ProstaScint® Scan: A method to determine whether or not cancer has spread to distant sites by using monoclonal antibodies. This test is especially helpful with patients who have been on hormonal therapy.

Prostate Capsule: The outer membranous covering of the prostate gland.

Prostatectomy: The surgical removal of part or all of the prostate gland.

Prostate Specific Antigen (PSA): A blood test that measures a substance manufactured solely by prostate gland cells. An elevated reading indicates an abnormal condition of the prostate gland, either benign or malignant. It is presently the most sensitive tumor marker for the identification and monitoring of prostate cancer.

Prostatic Acid Phosphatase (PAP): An enzyme produced by the prostate that is elevated (3.0 or higher) in many patients when prostate cancer has spread beyond the prostate.

Prostatitis: An infection or inflammation of the prostate gland that is treatable with medications.

Proton Beam Radiation Therapy (PBRT): A form of radiation therapy that utilizes protons as the source of energy (as opposed to X-rays or neutrons).

PSA: See Prostate Specific Antigen.

PSA Bounce (or PSA Bump): A rise in PSA level after first having a reduction in PSA after radiation therapy.

PSA Nadir: The lowest PSA value after a particular treatment.

PSA Velocity (PSAV): The rate of increase of the PSA level, expressed as nanograms per milliliter per year.

Radiation Therapy (RT): The use of high energy rays to kill cancer cells and malignant tissue.

Radiation Urethritis: Inflammation of the urethra caused by radiation therapy.

Radical Prostatectomy: An operation to remove the entire prostate gland and seminal vesicles.

Radiosensitivity: The degree to which a type of cancer responds to radiation therapy.

RBA or Relative Biological Effectiveness: A scale used to compare the intensity of radiation associated with various atomic particles.

Receptor: A cellular docking site that interacts with a specific protein or enzyme (called a ligand). The interaction typically leads to the synthesis of other substances such as proteins, hormones or enzymes.

Recurrence: Return of the cancer following remission or treatment intended as curative. Local recurrence indicates a return of the cancer at the site of origin. Distant recurrence indicates the appearance of one or more metastases of the disease.

Refractory: A term indicating that the cancer no longer responds to the current therapy.

Remission: Complete or partial disappearance of the signs and symptoms of the disease. The period during which a disease remains under control, without progressing. Even complete remission does not necessarily indicate cure.

Resection: The surgical removal of a part of an organ or structure.

Risk: The probability that a particular even will or will not happen.

RP: See Radical Prostatectomy.

RT: See Radiation Therapy.

Rx: The standard abbreviation for prescription.

Salvage Treatment: A medical term for "Plan B." It means a patient must undergo another form of treatment because the first therapy was not successful. Salvage therapy does not always work and often has a greater degree of complications.

Saw Palmetto: A nutrient extracted from the saw palmetto shrub, which is considered by some to aid the body's immune system.

Seed Implantation (SI): A minimally invasive procedure by which radio-active seeds are implanted into the prostate gland to destroy cancer. Also referred to as seeding and brachytherapy.

Selenium: A non-metallic element thought to be beneficial as a nutrient; it is often included in multivitamin supplements.

Seminal Vesicles: Glands that, like the prostate, support male reproduction. Fluid secreted by these glands regulates the consistency of semen.

Side Effect: A reaction to a treatment or medication, usually referring to an undesirable effect.

Sphincter: A circular muscle which contracts to close an orifice. The urethral sphincter squeezes the urethra shut, providing urinary control.

Staging: The testing process by which the extent and severity of a known cancer is evaluated according to an established system of classification. It is used to help determine appropriate therapy. See TNM Staging and Whitmore-Jewett Staging.

Surgical Margin: The outer edge of the tissue removed during a radical prostatectomy. The surgical margin may be "negative," indicating that no cancer is present and a better prognosis, or "positive," indicating that not all of the cancer has been removed.

Systemic: Throughout the body and affecting the entire body.

T-Cell: An immune system cell or lymphocyte that directs an immune response to malignant or infected cells.

Testes: Two male reproductive glands located inside the scrotum. The testes are the primary sources for testosterone. Also called testicles.

Testosterone: A male sex hormone chiefly produced by the testicles.

Thrombotic: Causing or relating to blood clotting.

TNM Staging: The most widely used classification system for evaluating the extent of prostate cancer. TNM refers to tumor, nodes and metastases. See Staging.

Transrectal: Through the rectum.

Transurethral: Through the urethra.

Transrectal Ultrasonography: See Ultrasound.

Transurethral Resection of the Prostate (TURP): A surgical procedure to remove tissue obstructing the urethra. The technique involves the insertion of an instrument called a resectoscope into the penile urethra, and is intended to relieve obstruction of urine flow due to enlargement of the prostate.

Tumor: An excessive growth of cells that is caused by uncontrolled and disorderly cell replacement. Abnormal tissue growth may be benign or malignant. See also Benign, Malignant.

TURP: See Transurethral Resection of the Prostate.

Ultrasound (Transrectal Ultrasonography): A painless, non-invasive diagnostic imaging technique using sound waves to create an echo pattern that reveals the structure of organs and tissues. It does not use x-rays.

Understaging: An overly low assessment of clinical stage at diagnosis.

Urethra: The tube that carries urine from the bladder and semen from the prostate out of the body through the penis.

Urologist: A physician who specializes in the diagnosis and the medical and surgical treatment of problems in the urinary and male reproductive systems.

Vasectomy: A surgical procedure to render a man sterile by cutting the vas deferens, thus eliminating the passage of sperm from the testes to the prostate.

Vasoactive: Causing the dilation or constriction of blood vessels.

Vesicle: A small sac containing fluid, as in seminal vesicles.

Whitmore-Jewett Staging: A classification system for evaluating the extent of prostate cancer. This system is less widely used for the designation of stage than is TNM staging.

X-rays: High energy radiation that can be used at low levels of intensity to make images of the body's internal structures, or at high intensity for radiation therapy.

QUESTIONS TO ASK YOUR DOCTOR

When first diagnosed with prostate cancer, a patient is likely to experience some degree of shock that may prevent him from absorbing the details of his case. Initially, the news of his condition may be all the patient can handle. But on a later visit, it is important for patients to obtain further information from the diagnosing physician. The checklist of questions below are intended to help the patient come to a better understanding of his condition, and to give him a foundation of knowledge for preparing to deal with his prostate cancer.

✔ How do you know I have prostate cancer?

✔ How far has the disease progressed?

✔ Before I decide on a course of treatment, what further tests should I have to determine the stage and nature of the cancer?

✔ What stage of prostate cancer do I have? How certain are you that my cancer is this stage?

✔ What are the treatment options for my stage of prostate cancer?

✔ Are there any treatment options other than those you have mentioned?

✔ What are the risks involved in each of the various treatments?

✔ What will happen if I am not treated?

✔ What treatment do you recommend, and why do you think it is best for me?

✔ Will the treatment that you recommend require hospitalization, or can it be performed on an out-patient basis?

✔ How many times have you performed this treatment in the last year?

✔ With the treatment you recommend, what is the rate and degree of impotence and incontinence among your patients?

✔ Does the site of the tumor in my prostate increase the risk of impotence or incontinence from the treatment you recommend?

✔ Is computerized planning sometimes involved in this treatment? Do you use such planning techniques? If not, why not?

✔ How will I feel during and after treatment?

✔ When will I be able to return to normal, everyday activities?

✔ When will I be able to resume sexual relations?

✔ What should I do if I experience erectile problems after treatment? Can you advise me or send me to someone who is an expert in the field?

✔ What should I do if I experience problems with incontinence after treatment? What can be done to treat incontinence? Is there an expert in the field you can refer me to in such an event?

✔ Will I need regular checkups to monitor the cancer and my response to treatment?

✔ What tests will be required for these check-ups, and what will they tell us?

✔ Are there particular warning signs for problems I should be aware of relating to a worsening of my condition or that might result from treatment?

✔ What do the different tests and treatments cost?

✔ How much of my medical expenses will my insurance cover and how much will I be required to pay out of pocket?

✔ Where should I go to get a second opinion?

✔ Do you use color-flow Doppler ultrasound as a diagnostic tool, or do you still rely on grey-scale ultrasound?

✔ Do you have the latest 4-Dimensional Image-Guided Intensity Modulated Radiation Therapy technology?

✔ Do you have the latest Dynamic Adaptive Radiotherapy (DART) technology for real-time imaging?

Questions To Ask Your Doctor Regarding Prostate Brachytherapy

✔ Do you perform modern transperineal brachytherapy with either ultrasound or CT guidance (in contrast to open free hand retropubic implants of the 1970s)?

✔ Do you believe in modern transperineal brachytherapy or do you perform the procedure only because of an increase of demands placed upon you by your patients? (Patients are advised to avoid physicians who are offering seeding only to keep up with patient demand).

✔ How many modern brachytherapy procedures have you performed and for how many years?

✔ How did you learn the procedure? Have you had years of hands-on experience or did you start practicing more recently after a two to three day seminar? (Years of hands-on experience is obviously much preferable).

✔ Is there a regional center where I might find doctors who have a greater degree of experience doing modern implant brachytherapy than yourself?

✔ How do you ensure that the seeds have been correctly placed?

✔ Following the procedure (immediately, but also several weeks post-implant) will you be doing an analysis to determine if the seeds are properly placed?

✔ What do you do if the seeds are not properly positioned?

✔ I understand that many doctors' "successes and complications" are typically quoted from the major implant medical centers, but what are your success and complication rates? Have these been published in the medical literature?

✔ What are your rates of rectal injury? What are your rates of urinary incontinence? What is your rate of erectile dysfunction?

✔ What is your success rate with patients having my stage and/or grade of disease?

✔ Following the procedure, will you be the doctor who directly follows my progress?

✔ Could you provide me with the names of other patients who you have implanted (preferably years ago with similar stage, grade and age)?

✔ What role do you think hormonal therapy has in the treatment of prostate cancer with brachytherapy with regard to down-sizing and/or sensitization?

✔ What are your specific guidelines for performing implant therapy? Who do you consider candidates for the procedure?

✔ If appropriate: Are you aware of the fact that I have previously undergone a TURP? Is a TURP a contra-indication for brachytherapy performed by an experienced brachytherapist?

✔ If no doctors have much experience doing implants locally and if I'm not able to leave the area to be treated, might I consider undergoing a procedure with which you are more experienced? (Patients should note that an inexperienced brachytherapist, like an inexperienced surgeon, is of little value and should be avoided. There is no reason why you should be on the early end of your doctor's learning curve, whatever his specialty may be. If there are no experienced brachytherapists in your area, and if travel is not possible, then you may achieve better results with an experienced surgeon if one is available to you locally.)

✔ If I choose to be treated by a more experienced doctor (out of town, for example), will you continue to be my doctor at home without there being any hard feelings?

✔ Do you use palladium or iodine seed implants?

✔ Do you combine brachytherapy with External Beam Therapy, and if so, do you have the most sophisticated EBRT technology (4D IG-IMRT with DART)?

✔ If you combine brachytherapy with External Beam Therapy, do you implant the seeds AFTER the external radiation treatments, like most leading physicians in the field?

✔ What can I do if my cancer comes back after brachytherapy?

REFERENCES

Al-rimawi M. Griffiths DJ, Boake RC, Mador DR, Johnson MA. Transrectal ultrasound versus magnetic resonance imaging in the estimation of prostatic volume. Br J Urol. 1994 Nov;74 (5):596-600.

Badiozamani KR, Wallner K, Cavanagh W, Blasko J. Comparability of CT-based and TRUS-based prostate volumes. Int J Radiat Oncol Biol Phys. 1999 Jan 15; 43 (2):375-8.

Badiozamani KR, Wallner K, Sutlief S, Ellis W, Blasko J, Russell K. Anticipating prostatic volume changes due to prostate brachytherapy. Radiat Oncol Investig. 1999; 7 (6):360-4.

Banker RL. The preservation of potency after external beam irradiation for prostate cancer. Int J Radiat Oncol Biol Phys. 1988 Jul;15 (1):219-20.

Bartsch G, Egender G, Hubscher H, Rohr H. Sonometrics of the prostate. J Urol 1982; 127: 1119-1121.

Bates TS, Reynard JM, Peters TJ, Gingell JC. Determination of prostatic volume with transrectal ultrasound: A study of intra-observer and interobserver variation. J Urol. 1996 Apr;155 (4):1299-300.

Bazinet M, Karakiewicz PI, Aprikian AG, Trudel C, Peloquin F, Dessureault J, Goyal M, Begin LR, Elhilali MM. Reassessment of nonplanimetric transrectal ultrasound prostate volume estimates. Urology. 1996 Jun; 47 (6):857-62.

Beyer D, Nath R, Butler, W, et al. American brachytherapy society recommendations for clinical implementation of NIST-1999 standards for (103)palladium brachytherapy. The clinical research committee of the American Brachytherapy Society. Int J Radiat Oncol Biol Phys. 2000 May 1;47(2):273-5.

Bice WS, Prestidge BR, Prete JJ, Dubois DF. Clinical impact of implementing the recommendations of AAPM Task Group 43 on permanent prostate brachytherapy using 125I. American Association of Physicists in Medicine. Int J Radiat Oncol Biol Phys. 1998 Mar 15; 40(5):1237-41.

Bice WS, Prestidge BR, Grimm PD, et al. Centralized multiinstitutional post-implant analysis for interstitial prostate brachytherapy. . Int J Rad Oncol Biol Phys. 1998; 41: 921-927.

Bittner N, Merrick GS, Wallner KE, Butler WM., "Interstitial brachytherapy should be standard of care for treatment of high-risk prostate cancer," Oncology (Williston Park), 2008 Aug;22 (9):995-1004; discussion 1006, 1011-7.

Blasko JC, Grimm PD, Sylvester JE. Palladium-103 brachytherapy for prostate carcinoma. Int J Radiat Oncol Biol Phys. 2000; 46: 839-850.

Blasko JC, Mate T, Sylvester JE, Grimm PD, Cavanagh W. Brachytherapy for carcinoma of the prostate: techniques, patient selection, and clinical outcomes. Semin Radiat Oncol. 2002 Jan;12(1):81-94.

Blute ML., "Radical prostatectomy by open or laparoscopic/robotic techniques: an issue of surgical device or surgical expertise?" J Clin Oncol. 2008 May 10; 26 (14):2248-9.

Cash JC., "Power against prostate cancer. Intensity-modulated radiation therapy and interstitial brachytherapy," Adv Nurse Pract, 2006 Sep; 14 (9):37-42.

Chan TY, Partin AW, Walsh PC, et al. Prognostic significance of Gleason score 3+4 versus 4+3 tumor at radical prostatectomy. Urology. 2000; 56: 823-827.

Cheng S, Rifkin MD. Color Doppler imaging of the prostate: important adjunct to endorectal ultrasound of the prostate in the diagnosis of prostate cancer. Ultrasound Q. 2001 Sep; 17 (3):185-9.

Crook J, Esche B, Futter N. Effect of pelvic radiotherapy for prostate cancer on bowel, bladder, and sexual function: the patient's perspective. Urology. 1996 Mar; 47 (3):387-94.

Dattoli MJ, Sorace RA, Cash J, Wallner K. Biochemical failure rates following combination external beam radiation and Palladium-103 boost for clinically localized high risk prostate cancer: 10 year results. Int J Rad Oncol Biol Phys. 2002 Oct; 52 (2) (Supp.1): 38.

Dattoli MJ, Wallner K, A simple method to stabilize the prostate during transperineal prostate brachytherapy. Int J Rad Oncol Biol Phys. 1997; 38: 341-342.

Dattoli MJ, Wallner K, Sorace R, Ting J. Planned extracapsular seed placement using Palladium-103 for prostate brachytherapy. J. of Brachy Int. 2000; 16, 35-43.

Dattoli MJ, Wallner K, True L, Cash J, Sorace R. Long-term outcomes after treatment with external beam radiation therapy and palladium 103 for patients with higher risk prostate carcinoma: influence of prostatic acid phosphatase. Cancer 2003; 97:979-83.

Dattoli M, Wallner K, True L, Cash J, Sorace R., "Long-term outcomes after treatment with brachytherapy and supplemental conformal radiation for prostate cancer patients having intermediate and high-risk features," Cancer, 2007 Aug 1;110(3):551-5.

Dattoli M, Wallner K, True L, Cash J, Sorace R., "Long-term prostate cancer control using palladium-103 brachytherapy and external beam radiotherapy in patients with a high likelihood of extracapsular cancer extension," Urology, 2007 Feb; 69 (2):334-7.

Dattoli M, Wallner K, True L, Sorace R, Koval J, Cash J, Acosta R, Biswas M, Binder M, Sullivan B, Lastarria E, Kirwan N, Stein D. Prognostic role of serum prostatic acid phosphatase for 103Pd-based radiation for prostatic carcinoma. Int J Radiat Oncol Biol Phys. 1999 Nov 1; 45 (4):853-6.

Davis BJ, Haddock MG, Wilson TM, Rothenberg HJ, Bostwick DG, Herman MG, Pisansky TM. Treatment of extraprostatic cancer in clinically organ-confined prostate cancer by permanent interstitial brachytherapy: is extraprostatic seed placement necessary? Tech Urol. 2000 Jun; 6 (2):70-7.

Davis BJ, Pisansky TM, Wilson TM, Rothenberg HJ, et al. The radial distance of extracapsular extension of prostate carcinoma: implications for prostate brachytherapy. Cancer, 1999; 85: 2630-2637.

Dicker AP, Lin C-C, Leeper DB, Waterman FM. Isotope selection for permanent prostate implants? An evaluation of 103Pd versus 125I based on radiobiological effectiveness and dosimetry. Semin Urol Oncol. 2000 May; 18(2):152-9.

Fang LC, Dattoli M, Taira A, True L, Sorace R, Wallner K, "Prostatic acid phosphatase adversely affects cause-specific survival in patients with intermediate to high-risk prostate cancer treated with brachytherapy," Urology, 2008 Jan; 71 (1):146-50.

Feigenberg SJ, Wolk KL, Yang C-H, Morris CG, Zlotechi RA, Celecoxib to decrease urinary retention associated with prostate brachytherapy. Brachy 2 (June, 2003) 103-107.

Feldman HA, Goldstein I, Hatzichristou DG, et al. Impotence and its medical and psychosocial correlates: results of the Massachusetts Male Aging Study. J Urol. 1994 Jan;151 (1):54-61.

Feleppa EJ, et al. Ultrasonic spectrum-analysis and neural-network classification as a basis for ultrasonic imaging to target brachytherapy of prostate cancer. Brachytherapy, 2002 (1) 48-53.

Forman JD, Kumar R, Haas G, Montie J. Neoadjuvant hormonal downsizing of localized carcinoma of the prostate: effects on the volume of normal tissue irradiation. Cancer Invest. 1995; 13 (1):8-15.

Gelblum DY, Potters L. Rectal complications associated with transperineal interstitial brachytherapy for prostate cancer. Int J Radiat Oncol Biol Phys. 2000 Aug 1; 48 (1):119-24.

Gelblum DY, Potters L, Ashley R, Waldbaum R, Wang X, Leibel S. Urinary morbidity following ultrasound-guided transperineal prostate seed implantation. Int J Rad Oncol Biol Phys. 1999; 45: 59-67.

Grimm PD, Blasko JC, Sylvester JE, Meier RM, Cavanagh W. 10-year biochemical (prostate-specific antigen) control of prostate cancer with (125)I brachytherapy. Int J Radiat Oncol Biol Phys. 2001 Sep 1;51 (1):31-40.

Han B, Wallner K. Dosimetric and radiographic correlates to prostate brachytherapy-related rectal complications. Int J Cancer. 2001 Dec 20; 96 (6):372-8.

Han B, Wallner K, Aggarwal S, Armstrong J, Sutlief S. Treatment margins for prostate brachytherapy. Semin Urol Oncol. 2000 May; 18 (2):137-41.

Howard A, Wallner K, Han B, Schneider B, et al. Clinical course and dosimetry of rectal fistulas after prostate brachytherapy. J Brachy Int. 2001; (in press).

Hu L, Wallner K. Clinical course of rectal bleeding following I-125 prostate brachytherapy. Int J Radiat Oncol Biol Phys. 1998 May 1;41(2):263-5.

Hu L, Wallner K. Urinary incontinence in patients who have a TURP/TUIP following prostate brachytherapy. Int J Radiat Oncol Biol Phys. 1998 Mar 1; 40 (4):783-6.

Hu JC, Wang Q, Pashos CL, Lipsitz SR, Keating NL, "Utilization and outcomes of minimally invasive radical prostatectomy," J Clin Oncol. 2008 May 10; 26 (14):2278-84.

Kagawa K, Lee WR, Schultheiss TE, Hunt MA, Shaer AH, Hanks GE. Initial clinical assessment of CT-MRI image fusion software in localization of the prostate for 3D conformal radiation therapy. Int J Radiat Oncol Biol Phys. 1997 May 1; 38 (2):319-25.

Khan MA, Partin AW. Management of high-risk populations with locally advanced prostate cancer. Oncologist. 2003;8(3):259-69.

Kim HL, Stoffel DS, Mhoon DA, Brandler CB. A positive caver map response poorly predicts recovery of potency after radical prostatectomy. Urology. 2000 Oct 1;56 (4):561-4.

Kleinberg L, Wallner K, Roy J, Zelefsky M, Arterbery VE, Fuks Z, Harrison L. Treatment-related symptoms during the first year following transperineal

125I prostate implantation. Int J Radiat Oncol Biol Phys. 1994 Mar 1; 28 (4):985-90.

Kollmeier MA, Stock RG, Stone NN. Urinary symptomatology and incontinence following post-brachytherapy transurethral resection of the prostate. Int J Radiat Oncol Biol Phys. 2003 Oct 1; 57 (2 Suppl):S439-40

Landis D, Wallner K, Locke J, Ellis W, Russell K, et al. Late urinary morbidity after prostate brachytherapy. (submitted 2002).

Lattanzi J, McNeely S, Hanlon A, Das I, Schultheiss TE, Hanks GE. Daily CT localization for correcting portal errors in the treatment of prostate cancer. Int J Rad Oncol Biol Phys. 1998; 41: 1079-1086.

Li Z, Palta JR, Fan JJ. Monte Carlo calculations and experimental measurements of dosimetry parameters of a new 103-Pd source. Med Phys 2000; 27: 1108-1112.

Ling CC. Permanent implants using Au-198, Pd-103 and I-125: radiobiological considerations based on the linear quadratic model. Int J Radiat Oncol Biol Phys. 1992; 23(1):81-7.

Ling CC, Li WX, Anderson LL, The relative biological effectiveness of I-125 and Pd-103. Int J Radiat Oncol Bio Phys, 1995; 32: 373-378.

Luse RW, Blasko J, Grimm P. A method for implementing the American Association of Physicists in Medicine Task Group-43 dosimetry recommendations for 125I transperineal prostate seed implants on commercial treatment planning systems. Int J Radiat Oncol Biol Phys. 1997 Feb 1;37 (3):737-41.

Maguire PD, Waterman FM, Dicker AP. Can the cost of permanent prostate implants be reduced? An argument for peripheral loading with higher strength seeds. Tech Urol. 2000 Jun; 6 (2):85-8.

Martinez A, Gonzalez J, Spencer W, Gustafson G, Kestin L, Kearney D, Vicini FA. Conformal high dose rate brachytherapy improves biochemical control and cause specific survival in patients with prostate cancer and poor prognostic factors. J Urol. 2003 Mar;169(3):974-9.

McNeal JE, Price HM, Redwine EA, Freiha FS, Stamey TA. Stage A versus stage B adenocarcinoma of the prostate: morphological comparison and biological significance. J Urol. 1988 Jan; 139 (1):61-5.

Meigooni AS, Sowards K, Soldano M. Dosimetric characteristics of the InterSource-103 palladium brachytherapy source. Med Phys 2000; 27: 1093-1100.

Merkle W. [Colour Doppler Transrectal 3D-Sonography of the Prostate–First Experiences]. Aktuel Urol. 2002 Jan; 33 (1):53-7. German.

Merrick GS, Butler WM. Modified uniform seed loading for prostate brachytherapy: rationale, design, and evaluation. Tech Urol. 2000 Jun; 6 (2):78-84. Review.

Merrick GS, Butler WM, Dorsey AT, Lief JH. Potential role of various dosimetric quality indicators in prostate brachytherapy. Int J Radiat Oncol Biol Phys. 1999; 44:717-724.

Merrick GS, Butler WM, Dorsey AT, Lief JH, Benson ML. Seed fixity in the prostate/periprostatic region following brachytherapy. Int J Rad Oncol Biol Phys. 2000; 46: 215-220.

Merrick GS, Butler WM, Dorsey AT, Lief JH, Totterd, Coram RJ. Influence of prophylactic dexamethasone on edema following prostate brachytherapy. Tech Urol. 2000 Jun;6(2):117-22. Int J Rad Oncol Biol Phys. 199; 43: 1021-1027.

Merrick GS, Butler WM, Dorsey AT, Lief JH, Walbert HL, Blatt HJ. Rectal dosimetric analysis following prostate brachytherapy. Int J Radiat Oncol Biol Phys. 1999 Mar 15; 43 (5):1021-7.

Merrick GS, Butler WM, Galbreath RW, et al. 5-year biochemical outcome following permanent interstitial brachytherapy for T1-T3 prostate cancer. Int J Radiat Oncol Biol Phys. 2001 Sep 1;51(1):41-8.

Merrick GS, Butler WM, Galbreath RW, Stipetich RL, Abel LJ, Lief JH. Erectile function after permanent prostate brachytherapy. Int J Radiat Oncol Biol Phys. 2002 Mar 15;52(4):893-902.

Merrick GS, Butler WM, Lief JH, Dorsey AT. Temporal resolution of urinary morbidity following prostate brachytherapy. Int J Radiat Oncol Biol Phys. 2000 Apr 1; 47 (1):121-8.

Merrick GS, Butler WM, Lief JH, Galbreath RW. Permanent Prostate Brachytherapy: Do Prostatectomy and External Beam Measure Up? J of Brachy Int., 2001 July-Sept, Vol. 17, 193.

Merrick GS, Butler WM, Lief JH, Stipetich RL, Abel LJ, Dorsey AT. Efficacy of sildenafil citrate in prostate brachytherapy patients with erectile dysfunction. Urology. 1999 Jun; 53 (6):1112-6.

Merrick GS, Butler WM, Tollenaar BG, Galbreath RW, Lief JH. The dosimetry of prostate brachytherapy-induced urethral strictures. Int J Radiat Oncol Biol Phys. 2002 Feb 1; 52 (2):461-8.

Merrick GS, Butler WM, Wallner KE, Galbreath RW, Lief JH. Long-term urinary quality of life after permanent prostate brachytherapy. Int J Radiat Oncol Biol Phys. 2003 Jun 1; 56 (2):454-61.

Merrick GS, Butler WM, Wallner KE, Lief JH, Anderson RL, Smeiles BJ, Galbreath RW, Benson ML.The importance of radiation doses to the penile bulb vs. crura in the development of postbrachytherapy erectile dysfunction. Int J Radiat Oncol Biol Phys. 2002 Nov 15 54 (4):1055-62.

Merrick GS, Wallner K, Butler WM. Management of sexual dysfunction after prostate brachytherapy. Oncology (Huntingt). 2003 Jan;17 (1):52-62; discussion 62, 67-70, 73.

Merritt CR. Doppler color flow imaging. J Clin Ultrasound. 1987 Nov-Dec; 15 (9):591-7.

Misraï V, et al, "Oncologic control provided by HIFU therapy as single treatment in men with clinically localized prostate cancer," World J Urol. 2008 Jun 26).

Mizowaki T, Cohen GN, Fung AY, Zaider M. Towards integrating functional imaging in the treatment of prostate cancer with radiation: the registration of the MR spectroscopy imaging to ultrasound/CT images and its implementation in treatment planning. Int J Radiat Oncol Biol Phys. 2002 Dec 1; 54 (5):1558-64.

Nag S, Sweeney PJ, Wienthjes MG. Dose response study of Iodine-125 and Palladium-103 brachytherapy in a rat prostate tumor (Nb-Al-1). Endocur/ Hypertherm 1997; 9:97-104.

Narayana V, Roberson PL, Winfield RJ, Kessler ML. Optimal placement of radioisotopes for permanent prostate implants. Radiology. 1996 May; 199 (2): 457-60.

Narayana V, Roberson PL, Winfield RJ, McLaughlin PW. Impact of ultrasound and computed tomography prostate volume registration on evaluation of permanent prostate implants. Int J Radiat Oncol Biol Phys. 1997 Sep 1;39 (2):341-6.

Nathan MS, Seenivasagam K, Mei Q, Wickham JE, Miller RA. Transrectal ultrasonography: why are estimates of prostate volume and dimension so inaccurate? Br J Urol. 1996 Mar;77 (3):401-7.

Nath R, Anderson LL, Luxton G, et al. Dosimetry of interstitial brachytherapy sources: recommendations of the AAPM Radiation Therapy Committee Task Group No. 43. American Association of Physicists in Medicine. Med Phys. 1995 Feb;22(2):209-34. Erratum in: Med Phys 1996 Sep;23(9):1579.

Nath R, Meigooni AS, Melillo A. Some treatment planning consideration for Pd-103 and I-125 permanent interstitial implants. Int J Radiat Oncol Biol Phys. 1992; 22: 1131-1138.

Peschel RE, Chen Z, Roberts K, Nath R. Long-term complications with prostate implants: iodine-125 vs. palladium-103. Radiat Oncol Investig. 1999;7(5):278-88.

Pierce LJ, Whittington R, Hanno PM, English W, Wein AJ, Goodman RL. Parmacologic erection with intracaverrnosal injection for men with sexual dysfunction following irradiation: a preliminary report. Int J Radiat Oncol Biol Phys. 1991 Oct; 21 (5):1311-4.

Pickett B, Fisch BM, Weinberg V, Roach M. Dose of radiation received by the bulb of the penis correlates with risk of impotence after three-dimensional conformal radiotherapy for prostate cancer. Urology. 2001 May;57(5):955-9.

Pound CR, Partin AW, Epstein JI, et al. Prostate-specific antigen after ana-tomic radical retropubic prostatectomy: patters of recurrence and cancer control. Urol Clin North Am. 1997; 24: 395-406.

Ragde H, Grado GL, Nadir BS. Brachytherapy for clinically localized pros-tate cancer: thirteen-year disease-free survival of 769 consecutive prostate cancer patients treated with permanent implants alone. Arch Esp Urol. 2001 Sep;54(7):739-47.

Rahmouni A, Yang A, Tempany C, Frenkel T. Accuracy of in-vivo assessment of prostate volumes by MRI and transrectal ultrasonography. J Comp Assist Tomo 1992; 16: 935-940.

Roach M, Faillace-akazawa P, Malfatti C, Holland J. Prostate volumes de-fined by magnetic resonance imaging and computerized tomographic scans for three-dimensional conformal radiotherapy. Int J Radiat Oncol Biol Phys. 1996 Jul 15; 35 (5):1011-8.

Roach M, Winter K, Michalski J, Bosch W, Lin X. Mean dose to the bulb of the penis correlates with risk of impotence at 24 months: preliminary analysis of Radiation Therapy Group (RTOG) phase I/II dose escalation trial 9406. Int J Radiat Oncol Biol Phys. 2000; 48: #2104.

Rosen MA, Goldstone L, Lapin S, Wheeler T, Scardino PT. Frequency and location of extracapsular extension and positive surgical margins in radical prostatectomy specimens. J Urol. 1992 Aug; 148 (2 Pt 1):331-7.

Roy AV, Brower ME, Hayden JE. Sodium Thymolphthalein monphosphate: a new acid phosphatase substrate with greater specificity for the prostatic enzyme in serum. Clin Chem. 1998; 17: 1093-1102.

Roy C, Buy X, Lang H, Saussine C, Jacqmin D. Contrast enhanced color Dop-pler endorectal sonography of prostate: efficiency for detecting peripheral zone tumors and role for biopsy procedure. J Urol. 2003 Jul; 170 (1):69-72.

Roy JN, Wallner K, Harrington PJ, Ling CC, Anderson LL. A CT-based evaluation method for permanent implants: Application to prostate. Int J Radiat Oncol Biol Phys. 1993; 26: 163-169.

Sauvain JL, Palascak P, Bourscheid D, Chabi C, Atassi A, Bremon JM, Palascak R. Value of power doppler and 3D vascular sonography as a method for diagnosis and staging of prostate cancer. Eur Urol. 2003 Jul; 44 (1):21-30; discussion 30-1.

Sethi A, Mohideen N, Leybovich L, Mulhall J. Role of IMRT in reducing penile doses in dose escalation for prostate cancer. Int J Radiat Oncol Biol Phys. 2003 Mar 15; 55 (4):970-8.

Shearer RJ, Davies JH, Gelister JS, Dearnaley DP. Hormonal cytoreduction and radiotherapy for carcinoma of the prostate. Br J Urol. 1992 May; 69 (5):521-4.

Sherertz T, Wallner K, Wang H, Sutlief S, Russell K. Long-term urinary function after transperineal brachytherapy for patients with large prostate glands. Int J Radiat Oncol Biol Phys. 2001 Dec 1;51(5):1241-5.

Shipley WU, Zietman AL, Hanks GE, Coen JJ, Caplan RJ, Won M, Zagars GK, Asbell SO. Treatment related sequelae following external beam radiation for prostate cancer: a review with an update in patients with stages T1 and T2 tumor. J Urol. 1994 Nov;152 (5 Pt 2):1799-805.

Singh D, et al, "Is there a favorable subset of patients with prostate cancer who develop oligometastases?" Int J Radiat Oncol Biol Phys. 2004 Jan 1;58 (1):3-10).

Sohayda C, Kepulian PA, Levin HS, Klein EA. Extent of extracapsular extension in localized prostate cancer. Urology. 2000 Mar; 55 (3):382-6.

Speight JL, Shinohara K, Pickett B, Weinberg VK, Hsu ICJ, Raoch M. Prostate volume change after radioactive seed implantation: possible benefit of improved dose volume histogram with perioperative steroid. Int J Radiat Oncol Biol Phys. 2000 Dec 1; 48 (5):1461-7.

Steinfeld AD, Donahue BR, Plaine L. Pulmonary embolizaiton of iodine-125 seeds following prostate implantation. Urol 1991; 37: 149-150.

Stock RG, Kao J, Stone NN. Penile erectile function after permanent radioactive seed implantation for treatment of prostate cancer. J Urol. 2001 Feb;165 (2):436-9.

Stock RG, Lo YC, Gaildon M, Stone NN. Does prostate brachytherapy treat the seminal vesicles? A dose-volume histogram analysis of seminal vesicles in patients undergoing combined PD-103 prostate implantation and external beam irradiation. Int J Radiat Oncol Biol Phys. 1999 Sep 1; 45 (2):385-9.

Stock RG, Stone NN, Kao J, Ianuzzi C, Unger P. The effect of disease and treatment-related factors on biopsy results after prostate brachytherapy. Cancer. 2000; 89:1829-1834.

Stock RG, Stone NN, Tabert A, Ianuzzi C, De Wyngaert JK. A dose-response study for I-125 implants. Int J Rad Oncol Biol Phys. 1998; 41: 101-108.

Stone RG, Ratnow ER, Stock NN. Prior transurethral resection does not increase morbidity following real-time ultrasound-guided prostate seed implantation. Tech Urol. 2000 Jun; 6 (2):123-7.

Stone NN, Stock RG. Prospective assessment of patient-reported long-term urinary morbidity and associated quality of life changes after 125-I prostate brachytherapy, J Brachy Int. 2003 March; 2 (1): 32-39.

Stone NN, Stock RG. Complications following permanent prostate brachytherapy. Eur Urol. 2002 Apr; 41 (4):427-33.

Sylvester JE, Blasko JC, Grimm PD, Meier R, Malmgren JA. Ten-year biochemical relapse-free survival after external beam radiation and brachytherapy for localized prostate cancer: the Seattle experience. Int J Radiat Oncol Biol Phys. 2003 Nov 15;57 (4):944-52.

Taira A, Merrick G, Wallner K, Dattoli M., "Reviving the acid phosphatase test for prostate cancer," Oncology, (Williston Park), 2007 Jul; 21 (8):1003-10.

Tapen EM, Blasko JC, Grimm PD, et al. Reduction of radioactive seed embolization to the lung following prostate brachytherapy. Int J Rad Oncol Biol Phys. 1998; 42: 1063-1067.

Teshima T, Hanks GE, Hanlon AL, Peter RS, Schultheiss TE. Rectal bleeding after conformal 3D treatment of prostate cancer: time to occurrence, response to treatment and duration of morbidity. Int J Radiat Oncol Biol Phys. 1997 Aug 1; 39 (1):77-83.

Tincher SA, Kim RY, Ezekiel MP, et al. Effects of pelvic rotation and needle angle on pubic arch interference during transperineal prostate implants. Int J Rad Oncol Biol Phys. 2000; 47: 361-363.

Wallner K, Blasko J, Dattoli MJ. Prostate Brachytherapy Made Complicated (Second Edition), Smart Medicine Press, Seattle, WA, 2001, p.4.6.

Wallner K, Lee H, Wasserman S, Dattoli M. Low risk of urinary incontinence following prostate brachytherapy in patients with a prior transurethral prostate resection. Int J Radiat Oncol Biol Phys. 1997 Feb 1; 37 (3):565-9.

Wallner K, Merrick G, True L, Cavanagh W, Simpson C, Butler W. I-125 versus Pd-103 for low-risk prostate cancer: morbidity outcomes from a prospective randomized multicenter trial. Cancer J. 2002 Jan-Feb;8(1):67-73.

Wallner K, Roy J, Harrison L. Dosimetry guidelines to minimize urethral and rectal morbidity following transperineal I-125 prostate brachytherapy. Int J Radiat Oncol Biol Phys. 1995 May 15; 32 (2):465-71.

Wang H, Wallner K, Sutlief S, Blasko J, Russell K, Ellis W. Transperineal brachytherapy in patients with large prostate glands. Int J Cancer. 2000; 90: 199-205.

Waterman FM, Yue N, Corn BW, Dicker AP. Edema associated with I-125 or Pd-103 prostate brachytherapy and its impact on post-implant dosimetry: an analysis based on serial CT acquisition. Int J Radiat Oncol Biol Phys. 1998 Jul 15; 41 (5):1069-77.

Willins J, Wallner K. Time dependent changes in CT-based dosimetry of I-125 prostate brachytherapy. Radiat Oncol Invest 1998; 6:157-160.

Wong YN, Mitra N, Hudes G, Localio R, Schwartz JS, Wan F, Montagnet C, Armstrong K., "Survival associated with treatment vs observation of localized prostate cancer in elderly men," JAMA. 2006 Dec. 13; 296(22): 2683-93. Erratum in: JAMA. 2007 Jan 3;297(1):42.

Yu Y, Anderson LL, Li Z, Mellenberg DE, Nath R, Schell MC, Waterman FM, Wu A, Blasko JC. Permanent prostate seed implant brachytherapy: report of the American Association of Physicists in Medicine Task Group No. 64. Med Phys. 1999 Oct;26 (10):2054-76.

Zaider M, Zelefsky MJ, Lee EK, Zakian KL, Amols HI, Dyke J, Cohen G, Hu Y, Endi AK, Chui C, Koutcher JA. Treatment planning for prostate implants using magnetic-resonance spectroscopy imaging. Int J Radiat Oncol Biol Phys. 2000 Jul 1; 47 (4):1085-96.

Zelefsky MJ, Leibel SA, Burman CM, Kutcher GJ. Neoadjuvant hormonal therapy improves the therapeutic ratio in patients with bulky prostatic cancer treated with three-dimensional conformal radiation therapy. Int J Radiat Oncol Biol Phys. 1994 Jul 1; 29 (4):755-61.

Zelefsky MJ, McKee AB, Lee H, Leibel SA. Efficacy of oral sildenafil in patients with erectile dysfunction after radiotherapy for carcinoma of the prostate. Urology. 1999 Apr; 53 (4):775-8.

Zinreich, ES, Derogatis LR, Herpst J, Auvil G, Piantadosi S, Order SE. Pretreatment evaluation of sexual function in patients with adenocarcinoma of the prostate. Int J Radiat Oncol Biol Phys. 1990 Oct;19 (4):1001-4.

APPENDIX E

CHARTING YOUR PROGRESS

It will be a great help to you to maintain a log of all tests and treatments you undergo during your battle with prostate cancer. This will accomplish several things. You will be able to supply on demand a history of your treatment to any physician you see. Following therapy, you will be able to personally keep an eye on your progress, and watch for any signs of recurrence. And rather than remain a mere bystander in your treatment program, you will be able to stay in charge of your own recovery.

The following pages include a Prostate Cancer Diagnostic Sheet, for recording the results of diagnostic tests, and a PSA Trend Chart, for visually charting changes in your PSA.

The Prostate Cancer Diagnostic Sheet lists the various diagnostic tests useful in the diagnosis and staging of prostate cancer. It is unlikely you will need to have all of these tests. However, proper diagnosis and staging will require that several of these tests be performed. Initial diagnosis is done with a digital rectal exam (DRE) and PSA blood test. If cancer is suspected, an ultrasound-guided biopsy should be performed.

Once cancer is detected, a battery of "staging" tests must be performed to determine the extent of the disease. The biopsy sample should be evaluated for differentiation and given a Gleason Score. The pathologist may also perform a DNA ploidy analysis. A bone scan is usually performed to check for spread of the cancer to the bones. Your doctor may also order a CT scan or MRI to visualize the extent and spread of cancer. Follow-up blood tests may include a second PSA test or a PAP blood test. In cases when the PSA is considerably elevated (over 20 ng/ml), a laparoscopic lymphadenectomy may be performed to see if cancer has invaded the lymph nodes. Before any test is performed, discuss its use and value in your case with your physician.

The PSA Trend Chart is an invaluable tool for the prostate cancer patient. For those engaged in "watchful waiting" to see if the disease progresses, the rate of rise in PSA values is a good indicator of the speed of disease progression. After treatment, a rising trend in PSA values probably signals treatment failure and recurrence of the disease. Be sure to discuss changes in your PSA, and the need for further tests or treatment, with your physician.

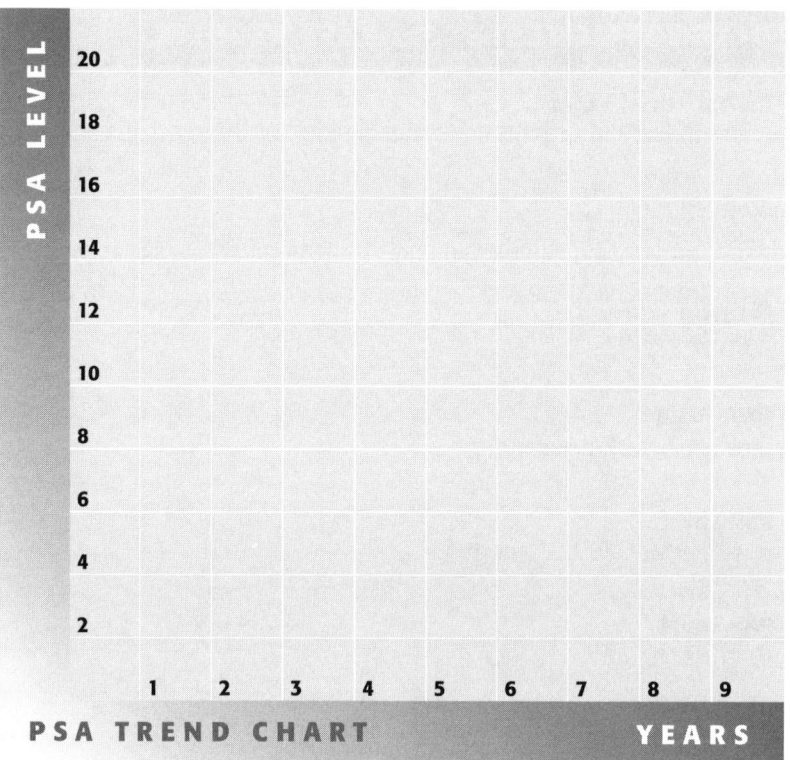

DIAGNOSTIC TEST	TEST RESULTS
Digital Rectal Exam (prostate size and shape)	
Biopsy (postive/negative)	
Gleason Score (value 2 to 10)	
DNA Ploidy (aneuploid, diploid, tetraploid)	
PSA Level (0 to greater than 1,000 ng/ml)	
PAP Level (0 to 100 ng/ml)	
Bone Scan (positive/negative)	
CT Scan (positive/negative lymph nodes)	
MRI (cancer confined to the prostate?)	
Ultrasound (cancer confined to the prostate?)	
Lymphadenectomy (positive/negative lymph nodes)	
Clinical Stage / Additional Notes	

NOTES

MY SUPPORT TEAM
Cancer Survivors, Doctors, Support Groups

Name: **Phone:**

E-mail:

Name: **Phone:**

E-mail:

Name: **Phone:**

E-mail:

Name: **Phone:**

E-mail:

Name: **Phone:**

E-mail:

Name: **Phone:**

E-mail:

Name: **Phone:**

E-mail:

Name: **Phone:**

E-mail:

Name: **Phone:**

E-mail:

Name: **Phone:**

E-mail:

Name: **Phone:**

E-mail:

Name: **Phone:**

E-mail:

Name: **Phone:**

E-mail:

INDEX

Y

Z

ABOUT THE
AUTHORS

Michael J. Dattoli, MD

Michael J. Dattoli, MD, is a board-certified radiation oncologist with more than 20 years of brachytherapy experience and has performed thousands of prostate implant procedures. Dr. Dattoli has successfully applied the same technology to other forms of cancer, including breast, GI, GYN, sarcomas and lung malignancies. He is a noted author and speaker in this complex field of medicine. He received his Bachelor's degree in Science from Vassar College and completed his Medical Doctorate at Mount Sinai School of Medicine in New York City. He completed his resident training in Internal Medicine at Westchester County Medical Center and Affiliates in New York and his Radiation Oncology resident training at NYU Medical Center and Bellevue Hospital. Dr. Dattoli also served as chief fellow in Brachytherapy and Radiation Oncology at Memorial Sloan-Kettering Cancer Center in New York and at New York Hospital-Cornell University Medical Center prior to relocating to Florida.

Jennifer C. Cash, MS, ARNP, OCN®

Jennifer C. Cash, MS, ARNP, OCN is an Advanced Registered Nurse Practitioner, Certified Oncology Nurse, Clinical Nurse Specialist and an integral part of the Dattoli Cancer Center Team. She is widely recognized for her particular expertise in all aspects of brachytherapy. Ms. Cash has an extensive background in Medical Surgical Oncology, Radiation Oncology and brachytherapy. She received her Bachelor's of Science degree and Master's of Science degree in nursing from the University of South Florida. She is a noted author and speaker on the subjects of brachytherapy, the most sophisticated radiation delivery systems, and hormonal therapies.

OUR MISSION

The Dattoli Cancer Foundation is a 501(c)(3) tax-exempt charitable organization, whose mission is

- ✔ to raise awareness of the wide-spread incidence of Prostate Cancer and the need for early and annual screenings;
- ✔ to provide information and support to men newly diagnosed with Prostate Cancer, as well as those with recurrent Prostate Cancer, and
- ✔ to foster research into better diagnostic tools and treatment options for Prostate Cancer.

Visit our Web site at: http://www.dattolifoundation.org

TO ORDER

To order more copies of *The Dattoli Blue Ribbon Prostate Cancer Solution,* write or call:

Dattoli Cancer Foundation
2803 Fruitville Road
SARASOTA, FL 34237

Individual or quantity trade orders: (800) 915-1001 or (941) 365-5599

ALSO AVAILABLE FROM DATTOLI CANCER FOUNDATION

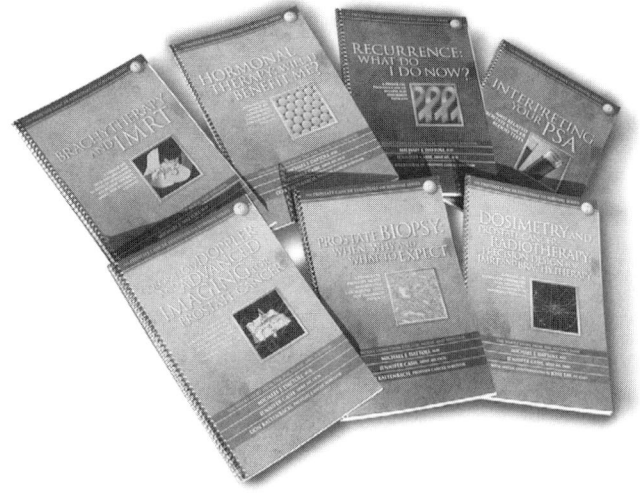

The *Prostate Cancer Essentials for Survival* booklet series is also published by the Dattoli Cancer Foundation. Some of the titles include:

1 *Brachytherapy and IMRT*

2 *Hormonal Therapy: Will It Benefit Me?*

3 *Recurrence: What Do I Do Now?*

4 *Interpreting Your PSA: And Related Prostate Cancer Blood Tests*

5 *Color-flow Doppler Ultrasound and Advanced Imaging for Prostate Cancer*

6 *Prostate Biopsy: When, Why And What To Expect*

7 *Dosimetry and Prostate Cancer Radiotherapy: Precision Design for IMRT and Brachytherapy*

To order copies of these currently available booklets and to find out when additional booklets will be released, please contact the Dattoli Cancer Foundation at (800) 915-1001.

DATTOLI
CANCER FOUNDATION

THE WARNING SIGNS OF PROSTATE CANCER

There are often no warning signs of prostate cancer. In some cases the following symptoms may indicate the presence of the disease. However, please be aware that these symptoms may also be due to benign conditions of the prostate, or other conditions entirely unrelated to prostate cancer:

- ✔ Elevated or rising PSA
- ✔ Abnormal Digital Rectal Exam
- ✔ Blood in urine
- ✔ Pain or difficulty urinating
- ✔ Increased urge to urinate, especially at night
- ✔ Hesitant or intermittent urinary flow
- ✔ Pain or discomfort in area of prostate
- ✔ Unusual and unexplained weight loss
- ✔ Continual pain in lower back, hips or pelvis
- ✔ Increased voiding urgency
- ✔ Inability to urinate
- ✔ Trouble having or keeping an erection (erectile dysfunction)
- ✔ Weakness or numbness in the legs or feet